Management and Competition
in the New NHS
(previously published as
The New National Health Service)

Chris Ham
*Professor of Health Policy and Management
and Director of the Health Services Management Centre,
University of Birmingham*

Radcliffe Medical Press
Oxford and New York

© 1994 Radcliffe Medical Press Ltd
15 Kings Meadow, Ferry Hinksey Road, Oxford OX2 0DP, UK

141 Fifth Avenue, New York, NY 10010, USA

British Library Cataloguing in Publication Data

A catalogue record for this book is available from the British Library.

ISBN 1 85775 013 6

Typeset by AMA Graphics Ltd, Preston
Printed and bound in Great Britain

To Matthew

Contents

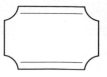

List of Figures, Tables and Boxes

Figures

Boxes

Tables

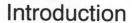

Introduction

The New National Health Service: organization and management was published in 1990 and provided a description of the reforms announced in *Working for Patients* and an introduction to the NHS (Ham, 1990a). This new book is a sequel and, in writing it, I have departed significantly from the original format. In part, this is because I have since collaborated in the production of a guide to the NHS (Ham and Haywood, 1992) which covers much of the same ground, and in part because it seemed more important at this stage to go beyond description and to seek to evaluate the reforms. The change of title reflects this different approach.

For the last six years I feel I have lived and breathed the NHS reforms. From Margaret Thatcher's decision to set up a review of the NHS in 1988, through publication of *Working for Patients* in 1989 and the anticipation of the reforms coming into operation in 1991, there can have been no more exciting time to be a health policy analyst. Add to that the experience of observing the 1991 reforms in action, and it has been an unprecedented period in the development of the NHS.

During those six years I have been involved in the process of reform in a variety of ways. Initially, at the King's Fund Institute, I worked with colleagues to analyse the options facing the government and to make an initial assessment of *Working for Patients* (Ham and others, 1989). This included a major study of the performance of health services in Europe and North America (Ham, Robinson and Benzeval, 1990).

Leading on from this, I contributed to the implementation of the reforms through my work at the King's Fund College with civil servants, health service managers and health care professionals. This work focused in particular on the development of the role of district health authorities as purchasers and it resulted in a series of reports on experience as it emerged in different parts of the NHS. These activities have continued since my move to the Health Services Management Centre at the University of Birmingham in 1992. Through a combination of research, consultancy and seminars I have maintained a close interest in the evolution of the reforms at all levels. In the course of a typical working week, this means spending three or four days in the field, working with purchasers, providers and others, both learning about what is happening in the NHS and passing on the benefits of this experience to those charged with making the reforms work.

In view of the rapid pace of change, I decided at an early stage to write up my observations and reflections on what was happening on a regular basis. The result has been a series of articles, papers and reports commenting on the reforms and trying to make sense of their impact. This book draws together many of the ideas from these publications but it seeks to go beyond them in two ways: firstly, it attempts to assess the impact of the reforms as a whole, not simply individual elements within them; secondly, and more ambitiously, it draws on experience gained since 1991 to identify the lessons that emerge and to suggest what needs to be done to take the reforms forward.

In writing the book, I have drawn on the results of my own work and that of other academics. This is not, however, the product of a traditional research project. Rather, it is an attempt to pull together data and intelligence from a wide variety of sources, to paint a picture of the background and development of the reforms, and to make an initial assessment of their impact. This task has not been made easier by the limited amount of research evidence available (the government always refused to support evaluation of the reforms), nor by the evolutionary nature of the changes. In time, some of the judgements will need to be revised in the light of further experience and as new data become available. Nevertheless, at the time of writing they represent my best assessment of developments so far.

I have received valuable support from my colleagues at the Health Services Management Centre, Anne van der Salm and Deirdra Keane, in the preparation of this manuscript. In addition, John Appleby prepared the figures for Table 1. I am also grateful to Philip Hunt, Chris Robinson and Angela Sealey of NAHAT for their comments on a draft of the book. I would like to thank my family for allowing me to steal the time to do the writing. The book is dedicated to Matthew (age 4) who has been especially understanding. It is a family joke that his first words were 'white paper'.

Chris Ham
April 1994

1 The Background to the NHS Reforms

The establishment of the NHS in 1948 was a bold attempt to make health services available to all citizens through a system of public finance and public provision. It was universal in its coverage and sought to be comprehensive in terms of the services that were available. To encourage the use of these services, there were no charges for treatment, at least initially, and it was the aim of the founders of the NHS to ensure that all necessary services were readily accessible in each area. The principle of equity was firmly enshrined in the structure of the NHS, meaning that care was to be provided on the basis of clinically defined need rather than ability to pay or other considerations. NHS finance was raised through a combination of taxes and insurance contributions, in the course of time supplemented by nominal charges for prescriptions, dental treatment and eye tests. A private health care sector continued to operate alongside the NHS but it remained a minor part of total health service finance and provision until the 1980s when it grew rapidly in response to the constraints imposed on the NHS.

The NHS in the 1980s

It was in the 1980s that the future of the NHS came under the critical scrutiny of Margaret Thatcher's governments. Administrative reorganizations in 1974 and 1982 sought to tackle weaknesses in the organization and management of health services whilst preserving the basic framework that had been put in place in 1948. In retrospect, these reorganizations can be seen as attempts to fine tune the integrated system of health service finance and delivery that was established in 1948. Figure 1 illustrates the structure of the NHS in England as it emerged from the 1982 reorganization. In this structure, district health authorities were responsible for running hospital and community health services and family practitioner committees administered the contracts of GPs and other independent contractors. The performance of district health authorities and family practitioner committees was supervised by regional health authorities and the Department of Health and Social Security. The result was a classic example of a centrally directed planning and management system

1

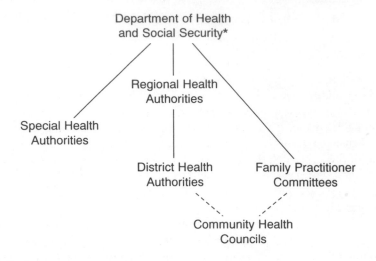

Department of Health
and Social Security*

Regional Health
Authorities

Special Health
Authorities

District Health
Authorities

Family Practitioner
Committees

Community Health
Councils

*The DHSS became the Department of Health in 1988

Figure 1: The structure of the NHS in England, 1982–90. (Source: Ham (1992a))

involving hierarchical relationships between different levels of management and increasingly sophisticated efforts to get the organization right.

The first significant departure from this approach came with the *Griffiths Report* of 1983. This left the structure of the NHS unchanged and instead sought to respond to evidence of variations in efficiency and the lack of attention to quality through the introduction of general management. In essence, this was an attempt to make the NHS more businesslike (Roy Griffiths was Deputy Chairman and Managing Director of the Sainsbury's supermarket chain) through the adoption of management methods drawn from industry. The Griffiths reforms reflected a wider set of changes in the public sector during this period designed to control the growth of public expenditure, ensure that there was value for money in the use of public funds, and improve the quality of public services.

Throughout the 1980s expenditure on the NHS continued to grow in real terms but at a slow rate. As the decade wore on there was a widening gap between the money provided by government and the funding needed to meet increasing demands from an ageing population and advances in medical technology. The impact of the funding shortfall became particularly apparent during the course of 1987 and was felt most

2

acutely in the hospital services (Ham, Robinson and Benzeval, 1990). In the autumn of that year, many health authorities had to take urgent action to keep expenditure within cash limits. This included cancelling non-emergency admissions, closing beds on a temporary basis, and not filling staff vacancies.

Behind these problems lay a funding system that failed to reward hospitals for treating extra patients. The so-called 'efficiency trap' was caused by the use of global budgets for hospitals that provided a fixed income regardless of the number of patients treated. This meant that hospitals were in practice penalized for productivity improvements because their expenditure increased in line with the number of patients treated but their income remained the same. In this situation, hospitals had little alternative but to reduce workload and cut costs when their budgets ran out.

The financial pressures facing health authorities were compounded by staff shortages. Media attention focused on Birmingham Children's Hospital where the shortage of specialist nurses meant that a number of children had their heart operations delayed. The parents of two of these children, David Barber and Matthew Collier, resorted to legal action in an attempt to bring the operations forward, but to no avail. Doctors added their voices to patients, demanding that something should be done. The British Medical Association called for additional resources to avert the funding shortfall and, in an unprecedented move, the presidents of the Royal Colleges of Surgeons, Physicians, and Obstetricians and Gynaecologists issued a joint statement claiming that the NHS had almost reached breaking point and that additional and alternative financing had to be provided.

The government responded in two ways. First, in December 1987, Ministers announced that an extra £101 million was to be made available to the NHS in the UK to help tackle some of the immediate problems. Second, the Prime Minister decided to introduce a far reaching review of the future of the NHS. This decision was announced during an interview on the BBC TV programme, *Panorama*, in January 1988, and it was made clear that the results would be published within a year. The Prime Minister established and chaired a small committee of senior Ministers to undertake the review, which was supported by a group of civil servants and political advisors.

In fact, this was not the first occasion on which a review of the NHS had been undertaken. A working party comprising representatives of the

Department of Health and Social Security, the Treasury, and the Health Departments of Wales, Scotland and Northern Ireland, together with two specialist advisors with experience of the private health care sector, had reported on alternative financing methods in 1982. As the Secretary of State at the time, Norman Fowler, explains in his memoirs, the government decided not to move away from a system in which the NHS was financed largely from taxation, on the basis of the working party's report. This was because other European countries were faced with similar problems to the UK and a centrally run and centrally funded health service like the NHS appeared to be most effective in controlling costs (Fowler, 1991).

In the absence of any specific proposals to change the basis of health service financing, Ministers pursued a policy of achieving greater efficiency in the NHS and encouraging the growth of private finance and provision alongside the NHS. The result was an expansion in the number of people covered by private health insurance schemes and in the role of private providers. By 1989, 13 per cent of the population in the UK was covered by private insurance. In parallel, the growth of private providers meant that by the end of the 1980s, eight per cent of all acute in-patients were treated privately and 17 per cent of all elective surgery was performed in the private sector. There was an even more rapid expansion of private residential and nursing home provision for elderly people and other vulnerable groups. Taken together, these changes meant that by the end of the decade private and voluntary hospitals and nursing homes supplied an estimated 15 per cent of all UK hospital based treatment and care by value (Laing, 1990).

The Ministerial Review

The Ministerial Review, initiated by Margaret Thatcher in 1988, offered an opportunity for alternative methods of financing and provision to be re-examined. The difficulty facing the government in this respect, as Norman Fowler indicates again, was that the NHS performed well when viewed in the international context. Total expenditure on health care, at around six per cent of GDP, was low by comparative standards, and yet for this spending the entire population had access to comprehensive services of a generally high standard. National planning meant that all parts of the country had access to health care, and a well developed system of primary care resulted in many medical problems being dealt with by GPs without the need to refer patients to hospitals. All this was achieved with only a small proportion of the budget being spent on administration (Ham, Robinson and Benzeval, 1990).

While problems clearly existed in relation to waiting lists for some treatments, poor quality of care provided for the so called priority groups, and lack of responsiveness to service users, they did not amount to a decisive case against the NHS. Rather, they indicated the need for a programme of reforms which retained the strengths of the NHS while the weaknesses were tackled. Indeed, for many of those who contributed to the debate, the most urgent requirement was extra money for the NHS to enable the changes that resulted from the *Griffiths Report* to be seen through. According to this school of thought, the key problem confronting the NHS was chronic and long term underfunding; there was nothing wrong with the structure of the NHS that additional resources would not overcome.

From this perspective, the control of health services spending exercised by the Treasury and seen by Norman Fowler as one of the strengths of the NHS, was in fact a major weakness in failing to deliver the volume of resources needed to fund the NHS to an adequate level. At a time when controlling public expenditure was an overriding political priority, it was not surprising that government Ministers were not persuaded by this argument, citing variations in performance across the NHS in support of their argument that existing budgets had to be used more efficiently before extra expenditure on the NHS could be justified (Lawson, 1992).

In its early stages the Ministerial Review focused on alternative methods for financing. This included looking again at the scope for increasing the role of private insurance and moving from tax funding to a social insurance system on the Western European model. However, this was soon superseded by an analysis of how the delivery of services could be reformed, assuming the continuation of tax funding. It was on this basis that ideas put forward by an American economist, Alain Enthoven, caught the attention of Ministers.

In a report published in 1985, Enthoven argued that an internal market should be developed within the NHS and this idea was elaborated by a number of right-wing think-tanks in their input to the Review (Enthoven, 1985). The contribution of Enthoven's thinking was later acknowledged by Kenneth Clarke who said that he liked Enthoven's idea of the internal market:

'because it tried to inject into a state-owned system some of the qualities of competition, choice, and measurement of quality that you get in well-run, private enterprise' (Roberts, 1990, p1385).

It was Clarke who played a major part in the final stages of the Review and who was responsible for presenting the government's proposals following publication of the white paper, *Working for Patients*, in July 1989 (Secretary of State for Health and others, 1989).

Working for Patients

In the white paper, the government announced that the basic principles on which the NHS was founded would be preserved. Funding would continue to be provided mainly out of taxation and there were no plans to extend charges to patients. Tax relief on private insurance premiums was to made available to those aged over 60, at the Prime Minister's insistence and against the advice of her Chancellor of the Exchequer (Lawson, 1992), but the significance of this was more symbolic than real. For the vast majority of the population, the NHS would continue to be the provider of health care and the government promised that access to care would be based on need. This was later reiterated by a future Secretary of State, Virginia Bottomley, in a speech to the British Medical Association:

> 'the government's commitment to the fundamental *principles* of the NHS has not wavered one jot. . . During the NHS Review, more radical actions were considered and rejected. They were thrown aside because they were incompatible with the sacrosanct principle of the NHS: that the care and treatment that the service provides should be available to any man, woman or child, on the basis of clinical need, regardless of the ability to pay' (Department of Health, 1993a).

The main changes in *Working for Patients* concerned the delivery of health services. These changes were intended to create the conditions for competition between hospitals and other providers. This was to be achieved through a separation of purchaser and provider roles: the creation of self-governing NHS trusts to run hospitals and other services; the transformation of district health authorities into purchasers of services for local people; the opportunity for larger GP practices to become purchasers of some hospital services for their patients as GP fundholders;

and the use of contracts or service agreements to provide links between purchasers and providers.

Fundamental to these proposals was that money would follow patients. This was intended to overcome the efficiency trap facing hospitals and to provide a stronger incentive than global budgets for hospitals to improve their performance. Ministers argued that a system in which providers had to compete for patients and resources would act as a significant stimulus to increase efficiency and to produce greater responsiveness to patients. The result would be a higher level of uncertainty on the part of providers about the source of their income but it was argued that this was necessary if the NHS was to tackle successfully the problems it faced.

These and other proposals were sketched in broad outline in *Working for Patients*, reflecting the speed with which the white paper had been produced. Subsequently, a series of working papers were published by the Department of Health containing more detail on different aspects of the proposed reforms. Together with the parallel changes to community care planned by the government, the proposals in *Working for Patients* were incorporated in the *NHS and Community Care Bill*. This was published in November 1989 and received the Royal Assent in June 1990, paving the way for the NHS market to come into operation from April 1991.

The debate about *Working for Patients* and the *NHS and Community Care Bill* aroused strong feelings on all sides (Ham, 1992a). Opposition to the government's proposals was led by the medical profession. The British Medical Association in particular opposed the introduction of market principles into health care. Organizations representing patients shared this concern as did bodies speaking for other professional and staff groups. There was more support for the reforms from managers and health authorities, although the timetable for implementing some of the changes was widely perceived to be unrealistic.

Figure 2 illustrates the organization of the NHS in England as it emerged after 1990. Unlike previous reorganizations, the structure did not change overnight and there was a progressive move away from the old to the new arrangements. Responsibility for overseeing the implementation of the reforms was vested in the NHS management executive working on behalf of Ministers. The management executive continued to be located within the Department of Health but increasingly it took on a separate existence from the policy divisions within the Department.

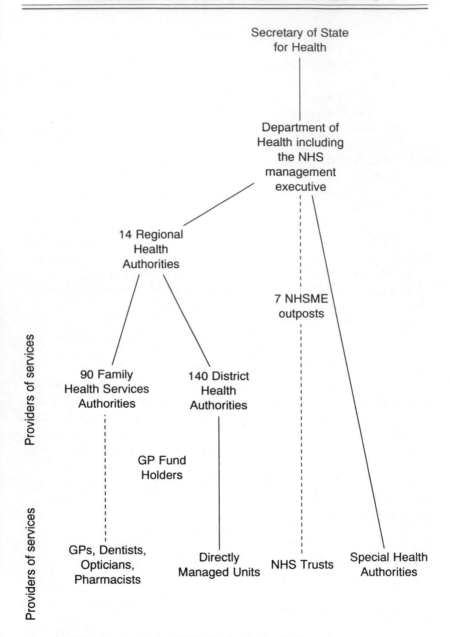

Figure 2: The structure of the NHS in England after 1990.

In this role, the Management Executive was used by Ministers to ensure that the reforms were implemented smoothly on the ground. The NHS Chief Executive, Duncan Nichol, assumed a higher profile as implementation gathered momentum, and attracted controversy in 1991 for supporting in public the policies of the government and appearing to criticize the opposition in the process. The NHS management executive worked increasingly with and through regional health authorities and sought to develop its role as the head office of the NHS. This was reinforced by the relocation of the management executive from London to Leeds in 1992.

Conclusion

The reforms to the NHS set out in *Working for Patients* were a response to acute funding problems that developed during the 1980s. Although the reforms in themselves did not tackle the long term underfunding of the NHS, they did seek to provide a way of ensuring that existing resources were used as efficiently as possible and that increases in productivity were rewarded and not penalized. More radical options for reform were considered and rejected during the Ministerial Review and it was for this reason that tax funding was retained. As Ministers emphasized, their proposals sought to preserve the founding principles of the NHS and to tackle the problems that existed by changes to the delivery of health services.

The logic behind this approach was that the NHS performed well when compared with other health care systems. To have proposed more fundamental reforms would have been to have put at risk the achievements of the NHS since 1948. Furthermore, from the Treasury's point of view, the great advantage of the NHS was its success in controlling overall levels of expenditure. Despite this, many of those involved in the NHS and a majority of the British public remained to be convinced that the proposals in *Working for Patients* would strengthen the NHS. The government's critics maintained that there was a hidden agenda behind the reforms and that the ultimate objective was to introduce a much higher level of private finance and private provision into the health sector. These are issues to which we return in the final chapter.

2 Implementing the NHS Reforms

The reforms introduced by the *NHS and Community Care Act* represent the biggest change to the delivery of health services since the inception of the NHS in 1948. Drawing on the ideas originally formulated by Alain Enthoven, it is often argued that the reforms involve the introduction of an internal market into the NHS. In fact, it is more accurate to use the phrase managed market. One reason for preferring this terminology is that competition is not confined to the NHS but also involves providers outside the NHS. Even more important is the fact that it has never been the government's intention to introduce a free market. Rather, the aim has been to graft some of the incentives that are often found in markets onto the structure of the NHS and to regulate or manage the operation of these incentives to avoid the problems of market failure.

The major developments in the implementation of the reforms are outlined in Box 1. As this shows, the reforms were implemented gradually over a period of years. *Working for Patients* contained proposals affecting almost all aspects of the NHS but the most significant elements of the reforms are:

- [ ] the separation of purchaser and provider roles;
- [ ] the creation of self-governing NHS trusts;
- [ ] the transformation of district health authorities into purchasers of services;
- [ ] the introduction of GP fundholding;
- [ ] the use of contracts or service agreements to provide links between purchasers and providers.

Taken together, the reforms involve a transition from an integrated system of health services financing and delivery to a contract system (OECD, 1992). They have proceeded in parallel with reforms of community care which are considered at the end of the chapter.

The Separation of Purchaser and Provider Roles

Before the reforms were introduced, district health authorities received a budget from regional health authorities to manage the hospital and

Box 1: The development of the NHS reforms.

1988

January — Margaret Thatcher announces Ministerial Review of the NHS.

July — Department of Health created following the splitting up of the Department of Health and Social Security. Kenneth Clarke appointed as Secretary of State for Health.

1989

January — *Working for Patients* published.

November — *NHS and Community Care Bill* published.

1990

June — *NHS and Community Care Bill* receives Royal Assent.

November — William Waldegrave replaces Kenneth Clarke as Secretary of State for Health.

1991

April — NHS reforms come into operation. The first wave of 57 NHS trusts and 306 GP fundholders is established in England.

June — The government agrees guidelines with the medical profession to avoid queue jumping by GP fundholders.

A green paper on *The Health of the Nation* is published.

1992

April — The Conservative Party is re-elected. Virginia Bottomley replaces William Waldegrave as Secretary of State for Health. The second wave of 99 NHS trusts and 288 GP fundholders is established in England.

July — A white paper on *The Health of the Nation* is published.

October — The report of the *Tomlinson Inquiry* is published.

1993

February — The government publishes its response to the *Tomlinson Inquiry, Making London Better*.

A review of functions and manpower in the NHS is announced.

April — The third wave of 136 NHS trusts and over 600 GP fundholders is established in England.

July — The functions and manpower review reports to ministers.

October — The government publishes its response to the functions and manpower review, *Managing the New NHS*. This includes the proposed abolition of regional health authorities, the merger of district health authorities and family health services authorities, and a streamlining of the NHS management executive.

1994

April — The fourth wave of 140 NHS trusts and 800 GP fundholders is established in England.

community health services in their areas. These services were directly managed by district health authorities who had a statutory duty to keep within budget and were responsible for maintaining appropriate standards of care. The cost of treating patients who used these services but lived outside the area was allowed for in the budget setting process. This was achieved by regional health authorities adjusting for the flow of patients across district boundaries and allocating resources to district health authorities accordingly. As a consequence, district health authorities were funded primarily to provide services in the hospital and community health services that they managed.

This was reflected in the way in which district health authorities carried out their responsibilities. For the most part, district health authorities were intent on expanding and improving health services in their areas and responding to the demands of those involved in service provision. It was this that led many researchers to conclude that the NHS was provider dominated and that district health authorities had been captured by providers to the detriment of other interests. The separation of purchaser and provider roles was in part intended to challenge provider dominance and to give greater attention to the needs of patients and the public.

It was also designed to break the strong link that existed between district health authorities and their local providers in order to encourage district health authorities to purchase services from other providers where this offered benefits to patients. In this way, providers would be put in the position of having to compete for contracts from purchasers. Instead of being funded to provide services in their hospitals, district health authorities are now allocated resources to buy services for the people who live in their area. This means that district health authority budgets are no longer adjusted for cross boundary patient flows but are based solely on the size of the population weighted for age, sex and other factors.

The architects of the reforms believed that competition would stimulate providers to increase their efficiency and to improve quality. This was to be achieved by creating a system in which money followed the patient. This principle was designed to overcome the efficiency trap which existed before the reforms in which providers were in effect penalized for treating more patients because their income did not increase in line with productivity. The obverse was that in the new system inefficient providers would be penalized if they were not able to attract contracts and resources from purchasers. These providers would then be forced to improve their performance or risk going out of business. This held out a quite different prospect from the old NHS in which hospitals only closed as a result of planned changes in service provision. In this respect, the logic of the reforms was inescapable: the introduction of competition in to a health service in which the budget was fixed meant that winners had to be matched by losers (Ham, 1989).

The separation of purchaser and provider roles did not happen immediately across the NHS. Rather, there was a gradual process of change in which initially the main priority was to clarify management responsibilities within district health authorities. This involved devolving responsibility for providing services to the unit level of management, leaving the staff at district health authority headquarters to take on the purchasing role. These changes resulted in a considerable reduction in the number of staff employed in district health authorities. This applied particularly to functions such as finance, human resources and estates, where there was almost complete devolution of staff and responsibility to units. As a consequence, a small core of staff remained at district level and they combined responsibility for purchasing with oversight of the performance of units.

A variety of management arrangements were put in place to achieve a separation of roles within district health authorities. These arrangements reflected the fact that district health authorities continued to carry statutory responsibility for directly managed units until they became NHS trusts and they therefore had to maintain an interest in the affairs of directly managed units. In this situation, district health authorities were characterized as 'holding on while letting go', having to ensure that directly managed units balanced their budgets and maintained appropriate standards of care while preparing these units to become self-governing organizations (Ham, 1990b).

Given that separation of roles was incomplete, and that district health authorities were responsible for any financial problems that occurred within their directly managed units, there was little incentive for district health authorities to move contracts from these units to other providers. To have done so would have created more difficulties than it would have solved because district health authorities would have had to deal with the consequences of budget shortfalls in their units. Any improvements in efficiency or quality achieved in this way would have been offset by the challenge of bringing capacity at local units into line with available resources.

It followed that initially competition was tightly constrained. It became clear that the development of a market in health services was contingent on a complete separation of purchaser and provider roles and the transfer of a majority of directly managed units to NHS trusts. Only in this way would district health authorities be able to become pure purchasers and reach independent decisions on where contracts should be placed.

NHS Trusts

The first NHS trusts were established on 1 April 1991. On that day 57 trusts came in to existence covering a range of services. These included acute hospitals, community services, mental health, learning difficulties, ambulance services and a combination of all of these services. Whereas *Working for Patients* had indicated that trust status would be available as an option for acute hospitals with more that 250 beds, in practice all services became eligible and it was quickly made clear that trust status was the preferred model for provider units. Accordingly, a further 99 trusts were established in 1992, followed by 136 in 1993. Most of the remaining units achieved trust status in 1994 at which point over 90 per cent of all services were managed in this way.

During 1992 the Department of Health made clear that it expected applications for trust status not to combine acute and community services. This reflected a concern that had emerged in London where there was evidence to suggest that in combined trusts budgetary deficits in acute services were tackled by taking money from community services. At a time when government policy was seeking to give greater priority to community services, establishing separate trusts for the management of these services was seen as a way of protecting their budgets. This policy was not, however, applied retrospectively, and trusts established in the first and second waves were not required to split acute services and community services.

Trusts were established on the basis that they would have a number of freedoms not available to directly managed units. These freedoms were of three types: financial, personnel and managerial. *Working for Patients* had indicated that trusts would have a degree of flexibility in borrowing money, enabling them to raise capital from private sources as well as the Treasury. In practice, this flexibility was largely illusory. Guidance issued by the Department of Health required trusts to borrow on the best terms available and in effect this meant borrowing from the Treasury. Furthermore, the amount that trusts could spend on capital developments was constrained by external financing limits set each year by the Department of Health. In practical terms, therefore, the financial freedoms of trusts were shackled by traditional public sector rules.

There was much greater freedom in relation to personnel where trusts were no longer constrained by national Whitley Council pay rates and terms of service but were able to negotiate locally with their staff. A number of trusts used this freedom to change the position of staff but in general movement in this direction was slow (IRS Employment Trends, 1993). Given the size of the NHS workforce, and the extent of the effort involved in renegotiating employment contracts, most trusts chose to make changes step by step and avoided any major departures from past practice. Insofar as change did occur, it involved a number of trusts making reductions in overall staffing levels. This is discussed further in the following chapter.

As a consequence, the management freedoms of trusts were more significant than the changes in the financial regime and personnel policy. In particular, the ability of trusts to manage their affairs as self-governing institutions, without having to report through district and regional health authorities, was an important innovation. The effect was to liberate managers and health care professionals to make much needed improvements in service provision. In this situation, trusts were held accountable primarily via the contracts they negotiated with purchasers rather than through the old line management relationship with the district health authority.

Alongside accountability through contracts, there grew up an arrangement whereby the performance of trusts was monitored by the NHS management executive. At first, this was done on a national basis, but the establishment of 156 trusts from April 1992 led to the creation of six (later seven) outposts of the management executive organized on a regional basis. Each outpost employed a small number of staff with the majority of the staff coming from financial backgrounds. The outposts were responsible for monitoring the financial performance of trusts, agreeing with them an external financing limit, and approving their business plans each year. Any suggestion that trusts should be held accountable through regional health authorities was strongly resisted by trust chairmen and chief executives who wanted to avoid being drawn back in to what they perceived as old style, bureaucratic controls. In order to protect trusts, the Secretary of State for Health wrote to the chairman of the Mersey Regional Health Authority in 1991 to emphasize that trusts did not come under the ambit of regional health authorities.

There thus emerged two kinds of agency at the intermediate tier of NHS management: management executive outposts, responsible for monitoring the performance of NHS trusts; and regional health authorities, given the job of overseeing the work of district health authorities and family health services authorities and managing the purchasing function. The future of the intermediate tier was itself reviewed during the course of 1992 and it was widely anticipated that regional health authorities would take management executive outposts under their umbrella. In the event, resolution of this issue was postponed until a review of NHS functions and manpower was undertaken.

District Health Authorities as Purchasers

The gradual establishment of NHS trusts, emerging like butterflies from the shell of a chrysalis, had the effect of slowing down the development of the new role of district health authorities as purchasers. Since much of the history and experience of district health authorities had focused on providers, there was a natural inclination on the part of managers working in district health authorities to continue to take a close interest in this side of the NHS. This was reinforced by the relative neglect of the purchaser role by Ministers and the management executive. In the early stages of the reforms, priority was attached to the establishment of NHS trusts and GP fundholders, and as a result it took some time before the full significance of the new function of district health authorities was recognized.

What support there was for district health authorities was focused nationally on *Project 26* (later renamed the *District Health Authority Project*) in the NHS management executive. This was a project which brought together 11 district health authorities from different parts of the country to share their experience of purchasing and to distil the lessons for dissemination across the NHS. In parallel, *Project 26* initiated a number of studies into how other district health authorities were taking on their responsibilities, and it commissioned a series of health needs assessment reports as a resource for purchasers. The result of all of this activity was a range of publications bringing together accumulated knowledge of purchasing (NHSME 1989, 1990, 1991, 1992).

Greater priority was attached to purchasing following the appointment of William Waldegrave as Secretary of State for Health and Andrew Foster as Deputy Chief Executive of the NHS management executive. Compared with their predecessors, Kenneth Clarke and Peter Griffiths respectively, both Waldegrave and Foster recognized the importance of purchasing and saw the establishment of an effective purchasing function as the key to making the reforms work. In particular, purchasers were seen as central to the successful implementation of the government's national health strategy. This emerged in a green paper in 1991 and a white paper, *The Health of Nation*, in 1992 (*see* Box 2). The strategy outlined a series of targets for improving the health of the population and Ministers made it clear that they saw purchasers as having the lead responsibility for delivering that strategy.

To help in the development of purchasing, £10 million was set aside nationally by Ministers in February 1992. This was reinforced in 1993, when the new Ministerial team at the Department of Health, led by Virginia Bottomley, gave a series of speeches in which they emphasized the significance of purchasing and maintained that purchasers had the major responsibility to drive ahead with the reforms. The lead in this area was taken by the Minister of State for Health, Brian Mawhinney, whose support for purchasing grew out of experience of bringing about changes in hospital services in London. At a time when the hospitals affected were universally critical of government policy, Mawhinney was impressed by the support he received from purchasers in London and their willingness to work with the government to achieve change. A further £4 million was earmarked nationally in 1993 as a resource for purchaser development.

One of the consequences of the establishment of NHS trusts was that proposals were put forward to merge district health authorities. There were a number of reasons for this, including the shortage of managers with skills in purchasing, the fact that some district health authorities were too small to form viable purchasing organizations, the greater financial leverage available to bigger district health authorities, and a desire to achieve coterminosity with other agencies, particularly family health services authorities and local authorities (Ham and Heginbotham, 1991). As mergers proceeded, many district health authorities sought to avoid the dangers of remoteness and insensitivity by setting up purchasing arrangements that were sensitive to the needs of small areas or localities (Ham, 1992b).

Box 2: The Health of the Nation.

Coronary Heart Disease (CHD) and Stroke
- to reduce death rates for both CHD and stroke in people under 65 by at least 40 per cent by the year 2000 (Baseline 1990)

- to reduce the death rate for CHD in people aged 65–74 by at least 30 per cent by the year 2000 (Baseline 1990)

- to reduce the death rate for stroke in people aged 65–74 by at least 40 per cent by the year 2000 (Baseline 1990)

Cancers
- to reduce the death rate for breast cancer in the population invited for screening by at least 25 per cent by the year 2000 (Baseline 1990)

- to reduce the incidence of invasive cervical cancer by at least 20 per cent by the year 2000 (Baseline 1990)

- to reduce the death rate for lung cancer under the age of 75 by at least 30 per cent in men and by at least 15 per cent in women by 2010 (Baseline 1990)

- to halt the year-on-year increase in the incidence of skin cancer by 2005

Mental Illness
- to improve significantly the health and social functioning of mentally ill people

- to reduce the overall suicide rate by at least 15 per cent by the year 2000 (Baseline 1990)

- to reduce the suicide rate of severely mentally ill people by at least 33 per cent by the year 2000 (Baseline 2000)

HIV/AIDS and Sexual Health
- to reduce the incidence of gonorrhoea by at least 20 per cent by 1995 (Baseline 1990) as an indicator of HIV/AIDS trends

- to reduce by at least 50 per cent the rate of conceptions amongst the under-16s by the year 2000 (Baseline 1989)

Accidents
- to reduce the death rate for accidents among children aged under 15 by at least 33 per cent by 2005 (Baseline 1990)

- to reduce the death rate for accidents among young people aged 15–24 by at least 25 per cent by 2005 (Baseline 1990)

- to reduce the death rate for accidents among people aged 65 and over by at least 33 per cent by 2005 (Baseline 1990).

Correspondingly, district health authorities and family health services authorities engaged in joint working of various kinds. In a number of regions, this resulted in the creation of health commissions and similar agencies. These agencies involved district health authorities and family health services authorities developing joint management arrangements, although these fell short of full integration as this depended on new legislation being passed by Parliament. Nevertheless, a study of joint commissioning by district health authorities and family health services authorities demonstrated that considerable progress had been made in developing comprehensive health plans, covering primary care as well as secondary care, and examining the use of resources in the round (Ham, Schofield and Williams, 1993).

In this context, the different approach taken by district health authorities and GP fundholders to purchasing in some parts of the country became a concern. With fundholders buying a defined range of services for their patients, and district health authorities purchasing the remaining services and the full range of care for the patients of non-fundholders, there was a risk of harmful instability if the plans of the two types of purchaser were not coordinated. In areas where district health authorities and fundholders worked together this was not a problem, but elsewhere it was difficult to see how the idea of a district general hospital providing a comprehensive range of services for a given population could be sustained when individual purchasers were intent on shopping around for the best deal for their patients. While Ministers emphasized the need for there to be shared purchasing between district health authorities and fundholders, the mechanisms to achieve collaboration were not always in place.

GP Fundholding

The first GP fundholders took responsibility for their budgets on 1 April 1991. On that day, 306 practices were established, involving GPs in England and covering seven per cent of the population. As with NHS trusts, more GP fundholders entered the scheme on an annual basis thereafter. By April 1994 there were 2,000 practices in the scheme in England involving 8,800 GPs and covering 36 per cent of the population.

The rules on GP fundholding evolved in the light of experience. Whereas *Working for Patients* had specified that only practices with

11,000 patients or more would be eligible to apply to become fundholders, this list size was reduced initially to 9,000 and subsequently to 7,000. At the same time, practices with fewer than 7,000 patients were encouraged to become fundholders by linking up with larger practices and by seeking the support of district health authorities and family health services authorities.

The range of services included in the fundholding scheme was also widened (*see* Box 3). To begin with, fundholding encompassed a limited range of hospital services, drugs and practice staff. In 1993, community services were added to the scheme, including district nursing and health visiting, chiropody and dietetics, and some services for people with mental illness and learning difficulties. On an experimental basis, a number of practices in different parts of the country tested the viability of purchasing other services, in a few cases taking responsibility for the whole of the budget for their patients.

In the early stages, one of the most controversial aspects of fundholding was the decision of some practices to set up private companies to provide services. This was a way of getting around the rules that practices were not allowed to use their resources to buy services from themselves.

Box 3: The growth of GP fundholding.

Originally, the scheme included the following services:

Hospital services: a defined range of elective operative procedures; out-patient services; diagnostic tests and investigations.

Prescribing expenditure: drugs and appliances.

Practice staff: the cost of employing staff such as nurses and receptionists.

In 1993 the following services were added:

Health visiting and district nursing.

Dietetic and chiropody services.

Mental health out-patient and community services and health services for people with learning difficulties.

Mental health counselling.

Referrals made by health visitors, district nurses, community psychiatric nurses and community mental handicap nurses.

In 1994, a number of pilot projects were initiated in which fundholders took responsibility for the full range of services.

In 1993, new guidance was issued forbidding fundholders from establishing private companies. As a *quid pro quo*, the rules were relaxed to enable GPs in fundholding practices to be paid for providing some services outside the scope of their existing contract such as diagnostic testing and minor surgery, subject to the approval of regional health authorities.

Research into the impact of fundholding demonstrated that GPs in fundholding practices brought about a number of changes in service provision. These included employing a wider range of staff in the practice, negotiating shorter waiting times for hospital services, switching contracts between providers where improved services were available, and reviewing prescribing patterns to obtain better value for money in the use of the drugs budget (Glennerster and others, 1992). On this last point, the evidence indicated that fundholding had proved more effective in curbing increases in prescribing costs than indicative prescribing (Bradlow and Coulter, 1993). This was of particular interest to the Treasury given the rapid increase in prescribing costs during this period and the absence of cash limits in this area of expenditure.

Supporters of the reforms cited these changes in service provision to argue that fundholders were at the leading edge of the reforms and were achieving greater success as purchasers than district health authorities. Against this, it should be noted that the practices included in the scheme initially were among the best organized and managed in the country, and the process of setting budgets in some cases erred in favour of GPs. Furthermore, district health authorities were constrained by their continuing responsibility for directly managed units and the emphasis placed by Ministers on the gradual and planned implementation of the reforms. In these circumstances, it would have been surprising if fundholders had not demonstrated greater initiative than district health authorities, particularly as their decisions attracted less media interest than those of district health authorities.

From the public's point of view, the most significant aspect of fundholding was the quicker access to hospitals enjoyed by the patients of fundholders compared with those of non-fundholders. Claims of a two-tier service surfaced very quickly after the introduction of the reforms and led to the government agreeing guidelines with the medical profession on priorities for treatment. These guidelines were framed in such a way as to be incomprehensible to most people. This was probably deliberate, enabling as it did a variety of interpretations to be placed on the guidelines.

In the light of this, it was hardly surprising that the British Medical Association was able to show, in a report published in 1993, that fundholders' patients continued to receive preferential treatment. The reforms made it inevitable that purchasing power would determine access to care rather than clinically defined need. Notwithstanding concerns that the principle of equity on which the NHS was based was being undermined, the British Medical Association dropped its opposition to fundholding, largely as a pragmatic response to the decision of an increasing number of GPs to become fundholders.

The process of setting budgets for fundholders was a matter of continuing debate. *Working for Patients* had envisaged that budgets would be based on a capitation formula. This was subsequently dropped in favour of a formula based on the use practices made of services in the past and their cost. Practices were also safeguarded against the cost of expensive patients by an arrangement under which fundholders were only liable for the first £5,000 of treatment for any one patient each year. This helped to ensure that GPs were attracted into the scheme and did not feel disadvantaged in the budget setting process.

One of the unplanned effects was that district health authorities, where there were a large number of fundholders and where budgets were set on the high side, found their own purchasing power significantly reduced. The inequity caused by this situation was reinforced by big differences in the amount of resources allocated to fundholding practices. In the first year of the scheme the average underspending among fundholders was four per cent although there were wide variations around this mean with some practices achieving six figure savings. While the rules laid down by the Department of Health barred GPs from benefiting personally from these savings, they were able to use underspendings to improve their premises and in the long term this did bring personal benefit. It is worth pointing out that a number of practices withdrew from the scheme or had their fundholding status withdrawn either because of loss of financial control or because the GPs involved felt their budgets had been set too tightly. For their part, some fundholders felt aggrieved when their budgets were reduced in line with the savings they had achieved.

In an attempt to overcome these difficulties, the Department of Health set in hand work to develop a capitation formula for fundholders and the early results were published in 1992. These results indicated that it would take some time before a capitation formula could come into effect fully, not least because there were problems in moving away from a budget based on historical practice patterns as this would mean big changes for some practices.

Alongside fundholding there emerged a variety of other ways of involving GPs in purchasing decisions. These ranged from GP involvement in district health authority purchasing, the development of locality-sensitive purchasing, and practice-sensitive purchasing (*see* Figure 3). A wide variety of initiatives were taken across the NHS and many GPs preferred to influence purchasing through these initiatives rather than by holding a budget directly. Partly because of this, it became clear that fundholding, unlike NHS trust status, would not become universal. Rather, there would be a mixture of methods for enabling GPs to influence purchasing decisions and no one model would apply in all places.

Contracts

NHS contracts provide the link between purchasers and providers. At an early stage, the government made it clear that contracts were not legal documents. In view of this, they are more accurately described as service agreements. The purpose of contracts, or service agreements, is to specify the cost, quality and quantity of care that should be provided. Contracts are made at the end of the purchasing process and set down in writing the range of services that NHS trusts and other providers have agreed to deliver to their purchasers.

Guidance issued by the Department of Health shortly after publication of *Working for Patients* envisaged that contracts would be of three main types: block, cost and volume, and cost per case. To begin with, most contracts negotiated by district health authorities were block contracts. These involved purchasers paying providers an agreed sum of money over a period of a year to deliver a defined range of services. Payments were usually made on a monthly basis and were tied to the provision of a certain workload during the year. For the most part, this workload was based on previous patterns of treatment and was expressed in general terms, for example the total number of in-patients, out-patients and day cases.

Cost and volume contracts involved purchasers paying an agreed price to deliver a specified volume of work. Any variation in the volume of work attracted additional payments or deductions as appropriate. Cost and volume contracts tended to be favoured by district health authorities placing smaller contracts and by GP fundholders. Cost per case contracts

Figure 3: Spectrum of options for GP involvement in purchasing.

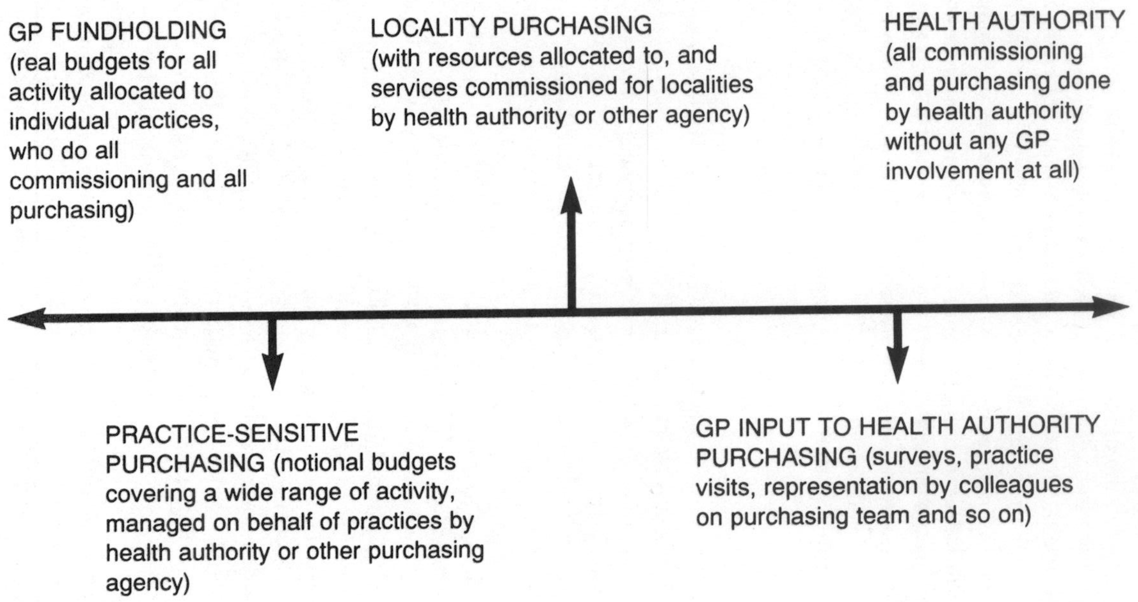

GP FUNDHOLDING
(real budgets for all
activity allocated to
individual practices,
who do all
commissioning and all
purchasing)

LOCALITY PURCHASING
(with resources allocated to, and
services commissioned for localities
by health authority or other agency)

HEALTH AUTHORITY
(all commissioning
and purchasing done
by health authority
without any GP
involvement at all)

PRACTICE-SENSITIVE
PURCHASING (notional budgets
covering a wide range of activity,
managed on behalf of practices by
health authority or other purchasing
agency)

GP INPUT TO HEALTH AUTHORITY
PURCHASING (surveys, practice
visits, representation by colleagues
on purchasing team and so on)

were even more popular among GP fundholders and were used by both fundholders and district health authorities to pay for the treatment of individual cases not covered by other forms of contracts.

One of the most controversial features of contracting was the use of extra contractual referrals. These were referrals made by GPs to hospitals which did not have a contract with the district health authority where the GP practised. If these referrals fell outside the terms of fundholding, the district health authority was responsible for approving them and agreeing to make payments. Under the rules laid down by the Department of Health, emergency extra contractual referrals had to be dealt with immediately and the cost met in full by the relevant district health authority. The same applied to tertiary referrals, that is referrals made by one consultant to another. On the other hand, elective extra contractual referrals had to be approved in advance by the district health authority following a GP's request.

This required district health authorities to establish procedures for handling extra contractual referrals and for determining how much money should be set aside for this purpose. In some cases, this involved negotiating with GPs as to whether the referral was necessary. In other cases, particularly where budgets were tight, it meant refusing to approve extra contractual referrals or delaying them until the following financial year, thereby limiting the freedom of choice of GPs and patients. In practice, difficulties of this kind arose only in a small proportion of cases, but it was nevertheless an issue on which many GPs and patients felt strongly. The administration of extra contractual referrals was also costly and time consuming.

As purchasers and providers gained experience of contracting, the Department of Health encouraged movement away from simple block contracts to more sophisticated arrangements. This included making use of contracts for more than a period of one year, specifying floors and ceilings for the workload to be performed, and introducing a wide range of incentives and penalties into contracts. While some progress was made in all of these areas, the development of more sophisticated contracts was hampered by weaknesses in both information and costing systems.

There was also a reluctance on the part of some purchasers to assume the risks involved in more sophisticated contracts. Block contracts were undoubtedly a crude tool but they at least had the virtue from a purchaser's point of view of controlling expenditure. The greater use of contracts in which planned increases in activity triggered additional payments for providers created more uncertainty for purchasers and the risk that their budgets would be overspent. Given the absence of reliable information on case mix, there was also a danger that unscrupulous providers would 'game' the system to their advantage by maximizing the throughput of simple cases at the expense of those that were more complex. In view of the lack of tried and tested methods for monitoring contract compliance, many purchasers were reluctant to expose themselves to this danger.

The difficulty this created for providers was that increases in activity were not rewarded with increases in income. In other words, the efficiency trap which gave rise to the NHS reforms continued to cause problems. Providers that fulfilled their contracts ahead of schedule were forced to postpone elective admissions until their new contracts came into operation. As a number of observers pointed out, far from money following the patients, the patients were required to follow the money associated with block contracts (Ham, 1992c).

In this situation, the incentives to improve performance that the reforms were supposed to introduce were not much in evidence. The response of Ministers was to urge providers to manage their workload more effectively throughout the year and to ensure that clinicians were involved fully in contract negotiations. This achieved some success in avoiding hospitals having to stop admissions part way through the year but the underlying problem of a health service in which there was a mismatch between resource allocation and activity remained. Despite these problems, there were a number of examples of good practice in contracting. These were highlighted in a report from the management executive published in 1993. Examples drawn from the report are displayed in Box 4.

One of the concerns expressed at the inception of the reforms was that quality would be sacrificed by purchasers in the pursuit of increased activity and lower prices. Evidence from the use of contracts indicates that a wide range of quality standards were specified by purchasers, covering such issues as waiting times, patient satisfaction, and a requirement to undertake medical audit. Much less attention was paid to standards of clinical quality. This reflects largely the absence of data on clinical quality and the difficulty of comparing providers on a consistent basis. Publication of the *Patient's Charter* in October 1991 (*see* Box 5) ensured that the emphasis continued to be placed on issues of access and patient convenience. The planned publication of league tables of the

Box 4: Good practice in contracting.

Salford District Health Authority was planning to use 'block plus' contracts with its top ten providers in 1994/95. These contracts would have floor and ceiling levels within five per cent of the target volume of activity. Additional payments would be made at marginal costs.

The West Midlands Regional Health Authority and its district health authorities used a regional specialties agency to negotiate contracts for regional specialties. The rationale for this is that specialties with high costs and low volumes require a different approach from other services. The agency acts on behalf of all district health authorities in the region to purchase regional specialty services from designated units.

Four health commissions in the Wessex region collaborated over the production of a common set of quality specifications for inclusion in contracts. This included an approach to monitoring, involving annual visits to all providers, quality reports and information from GPs.

The Mersey Regional Health Authority developed a system of incentives to reduce waiting times for treatment. Bonus payments are made to providers who achieve the regional target of no patient waiting longer than 12 months. Where a provider fails to meet the target, the district health authority is encouraged to claw back waiting time funds and invest them elsewhere.

---

performance of providers based on the *Patient's Charter* is likely to mean that these aspects of quality will receive even greater prominence in future.

A number of issues relating to contracts were reviewed in the first reports to be published by the Clinical Standards Advisory Group. The government agreed to set up this Group during the debate on the *NHS and Community Care Bill*, in response to representations from the medical profession that there should be an independent source of expert advice to the UK Health Ministers and the NHS on standards of clinical care. Initially, the Clinical Standards Advisory Group reviewed arrangements made for four services: neonatal intensive care, cystic fibrosis, childhood leukaemia, and coronary artery bypass grafting and angiography. In a wide ranging review, the Group concluded that contracting was taking place in a rudimentary fashion, that contracts were too crude an instrument to be used in purchasing specialized services, and professional staff had been insufficiently involved in the preparation of contracts. The Group also argued that individual district health authorities did not always have the expertise needed to purchase these specialist services and

Box 5: The Patient's Charter.

There are **ten rights** included in the *Patient's Charter*. These are:

- to receive health care on the basis of clinical need, regardless of ability to pay;
- to be registered with a GP;
- to receive emergency medical care at any time through a GP or through the emergency ambulance service and hospital accident and emergency department;
- to be referred to a consultant, acceptable to a patient, when a GP thinks this necessary and to be referred for a second opinion if a patient and GP agree this is desirable;
- to be given a clear explanation of any treatment proposed, including any risks and alternatives;
- to have access to health records, and to know that those working for the NHS are under a legal duty to keep their contents confidential;
- to choose whether or not to take part in medical research or medical student training;
- to be given detailed information on local health services, including quality standards and maximum waiting times;
- to be guaranteed admission for treatment by a specific date no later than two years from the day when a patient is placed on a waiting list;
- to have any complaint about NHS services investigated and to receive a full and prompt written reply from the chief executive or general manager.

collaboration between health authorities might be needed in future. The Group concluded that issues concerned with clinical quality had been largely ignored (Clinical Standards Advisory Group, 1993). In response, the Department of Health issued revised guidance to health authorities on contracting for specialist services.

Community Care

In parallel with the reforms to the NHS, the government introduced major changes to the financing and delivery of community care. These changes stemmed from the white paper, *Caring for People*, which was itself a response to a report prepared by Sir Roy Griffiths in 1988. Both documents acknowledged that progress in developing services in the community for vulnerable groups, such as the frail elderly and the mentally ill, had been patchy. Furthermore, there was an incentive to admit people to residential care in the community, for example nursing homes, rather than to provide support in people's own homes. This was because residential care was funded through the social security budget and had to be provided to individuals who met the requirements for income support. The existence of this entitlement meant that expenditure on this part of the social security budget increased rapidly during the 1980s. The reforms set out in *Caring for People* were intended to halt the rise in expenditure, remove the incentive to use residential care, and ensure that a wider range of services was available to those in need.

The provisions of *Caring for People* were incorporated in the *NHS and Community Care Act* of 1990. The Act gave local authorities the lead responsibility for community care and their role was that of enablers rather than direct service providers. Local authorities were required to prepare community care plans in association with health authorities and other agencies. They were also given additional resources to enable them to discharge their responsibilities. Most of these resources involved the transfer of funds from the social security budget. The government made it clear that it expected these funds to be used primarily to buy services from providers in the independent sector rather than to fund direct provision by local authorities. This meant that a community care market began to grow alongside the NHS market based on a separation of purchaser and provider roles, the use of contracts, and the emergence of a mixed economy of care.

The original intention was that the changes to community care would be implemented at the same time as the reforms of the NHS. In the event, the government delayed implementing the transfer of funds to local authorities until 1993 because of difficulties that had arisen over the community charge, or poll tax. Local authorities used the intervening period to prepare themselves for the new arrangements, including making provision for the assessment of individuals' needs for care. The principal responsibility for needs assessment rested with care managers employed by local authorities. Care managers were expected to work with GPs and other colleagues from the NHS to determine what services were required.

In 1993/94, £399 million was transferred from the social security budget to local authorities as the first stage in implementing the community care reforms. These resources were ring-fenced to ensure that they were indeed used for this purpose. At the same time, the government provided a further £140 million, in recognition of the additional costs that local authorities incurred as a result of the changes. The associations representing local authorities argued that these sums fell short of what was required and would mean that not all needs could be met. This gave rise to concerns that some individuals might receive no services at all, even though they had been assessed as in need, while others would be cared for in inappropriate settings. In particular, health authorities feared that acute hospital beds might be blocked by elderly people ready to be discharged but for whom no alternative services were available.

In the broader context, the community care reforms highlighted the importance of priority setting or rationing. The shift from a funding system in which individuals were entitled to income support for residential care to one in which local authorities determined who obtained access to services by allocating a fixed budget, represented a fundamental change of approach. While it was widely recognized that there was scope for obtaining better value for money within existing budgets, there were also doubts about the adequacy of overall levels of funding in view of the increasing demands presented by an ageing population. In this respect, local authorities were faced with many of the same dilemmas as health authorities.

One of the risks that this gave rise to was that of cost shifting or buck passing. Put another way, faced with more needs than it was possible to accommodate within available resources, health authorities and local authorities might be tempted to transfer responsibility to each other. This risk was accentuated by the lack of clear definitions of health care on the one hand and community care on the other. In this situation, it was argued that health authorities and local authorities might adopt an increasingly narrow interpretation of their own responsibilities, leaving vulnerable clients and patients to fall between the two.

In trying to avoid this, authorities in many parts of the country took the initiative to establish joint commissioning arrangements. These arrangements often built on earlier experience of joint planning and joint finance, and sought to ensure that there was a consistent approach between different agencies. In a number of places, there was interest not only in joint planning and needs assessment but also the pooling of resources for particular services or care groups. The development of joint commissioning suggested that in the longer term the division of responsibilities between the NHS and local government might be reviewed, with either local authorities taking responsibility for the commissioning of health services or the commissioning of social services passing to the NHS.

Conclusion

In this chapter, we have traced the development of the key elements in the NHS reforms in the period after 1991. We have shown how purchaser and provider roles were gradually separated with district health authorities taking on responsibility for purchasing and NHS trust status becoming the model of choice for provider units. An increasing number of GP practices entered the fundholding scheme while non-fundholding GPs were involved in purchasing through a variety of mechanisms. Contracts, or service agreements, provided the link between purchasers and providers and became increasingly sophisticated with time.

The question that arises from these developments is what was the impact on patients and service providers? Did the reforms achieve the improvements in services that were intended? Or was there an expansion of management costs, as the government's critics argued, with few if any benefits for patients? And what impact did competition have on the delivery of services? These are the questions addressed in the next chapter.

3 | The Impact of the NHS Reforms

In an article for *The Guardian* in September 1992 I wrote:

The NHS reforms are about to enter their third and most risky phase. This phase can be likened to the transition from childhood to adolescence. It follows a period of growth and development in which an infant that barely survived the trauma of premature birth has become steadily more mature and confident.

Many of the difficulties encountered during childhood can be attributed to the abrupt and untimely way in which gestation was brought to an end. The midwife, Margaret Thatcher, insisted that the baby should be delivered within one year of conception. As a consequence, developments which should have occurred in the womb in practice took place in the first year of life.

It was in this period, following publication of the white paper, *Working for Patients*, that the offspring began to take shape. Many of the features that were barely discernible at birth emerged more clearly and by the time the white paper had passed into law it was possible to see the nature of the being that had been created. At this point, in the summer of 1990, the second phase started.

In this phase, there has been a period of sustained growth, and the baby has become a child. The child has acquired skills such as walking and talking and an identifiable personality of its own. It has even been known to disobey its parents on occasion. This has resulted in disciplinary action. The controls that are being imposed are so tight that the neighbours have sometimes wondered whether the child still lives at home.

But with the election out of the way, and the autumn approaching, the infant prodigy has started to try out his newly acquired skills. This has resulted in demands for greater freedom and even a request to stay with friends overnight. The current foster parents (the natural father has since moved to administer similar treatment to teachers and the police) are understandably anxious about these requests and are not yet sure that the child is sufficiently mature to be allowed this degree of latitude. At the same time, they realize that it won't be long before he leaves home for good. They know that independence in the longer term may be more easily achieved if risks are taken now.

It is these issues that the occupants of Richmond House agonize over. Having survived a difficult first year, and a sheltered childhood, should their offspring be given greater freedom? If he is, won't this result in mistakes which unsympathetic members of the family will blame on the parents? And .wouldn't it be easier to protect the child from an increasingly hostile environment by maintaining its growth sheltered from the slings and arrows of fortune? These questions are as yet unresolved, but if the parents don't make up their minds soon the flowering adolescent may take matters into his own hands with unpredictable consequences for all.

To complicate the decision, in the same household there is an adopted child who has been told that she can leave home in April 1993. Like her sibling, she has suffered a series of setbacks, and was originally told she would be given her independence in 1991. But the adults thought it better to wait until her inheritance had been sorted out and for this reason there has been a delay. In the meantime, the two children have been encouraged to play together in the hope that they will become friends for life.

This metaphor may not exactly fit developments in the NHS (and its close relation, community care) but it highlights many of the dilemmas facing the current ministerial team. Above all, the metaphor illustrates that the key decision is whether to take some risks, knowing that mistakes will be made along the way, or to play safe, in the awareness that this strategy is also fraught with difficulties. It is a decision with which parents are familiar and which calls for careful judgment at a crucial stage in the life-cycle of change.

For Virginia Bottomley, a parent herself, the central choice is about the pace of development. Having taken over responsibility for the NHS and community care reforms from her predecessors, she is not in a position to question the direction of change. The most important decision at this stage is how quickly the reforms should proceed and the degree of freedom that should be allowed to local agencies in taking the reforms forward. In pondering this question, the Health Secretary is under pressure from her supporters to allow much greater competition in the internal health care market than has hitherto been permitted. She is also aware that many of those involved in running the NHS at a local level are keen to try out their new freedoms and functions and are increasingly impatient at the constraints imposed from above. And, to vary the metaphor, having let the genie out of the bottle, it will be difficult to squeeze it back in.

Nevertheless, ministers are in a position to shape the framework within which competition occurs, not least by insisting that the

market should be managed rather than left to the independent decisions of health authorities and NHS trusts. In this way it ought to be
possible to relax some of the controls exercised by Ministers while
ensuring that the process of change remains orderly. It is here that
the role of regional health authorities is crucial. Ministers cannot
direct the development of health services and community care from
Whitehall and they must rely on an intermediate tier to act on their
behalf.

Yet as things stand, the responsibilities of the intermediate tier
are divided between regional health authorities and outposts of the
NHS management executive in a bureaucratic confusion of the
worst kind.

Faced with this confusion, Ministers need to act quickly. Above
all, there must be the capacity at regional level to take a coherent
view of the internal market and to manage competition in a way
which balances greater freedom for health authorities and NHS
trusts with an appropriate degree of regulation.

This is one of the issues that Mrs Bottomley has been considering
over the summer, and an early decision is needed. If a single agency
charged with managing the market, is not established at the regional level, then the reforms could become discredited. The potential
benefits in terms of greater efficiency and enhanced responsiveness
to patients, which have already started to emerge, will not be real-
ized.

The urgency of this issue is highlighted by the difficulties faced by
hospitals in London which have had to cut back their services
because they have not attracted sufficient contracts. Competition is
already starting to have an impact, but there is no guarantee that
market forces alone will produce an appropriate pattern of services.

The reality is that the market has to be regulated by a strategic
body in a position to preserve the founding principles of the NHS at
a time when new values are increasingly evident.

To return to the original metaphor, the adolescent may find him-
self in trouble if clear expectations are not established about the limits of independent action and standards of acceptable behaviour. If
this were to happen, it would reflect badly not only on the offspring
but also on the parents (Ham 1992a).

There are two points about this article which are central to an analysis of
the impact of the NHS reforms. First, carrying out the reforms has
involved a process of development in which their true nature has become
clear only in the course of implementation. Second, at the heart of the

reforms is the attempt to introduce a managed market in healthcare. A crucial judgement for Ministers is whether competition should be allowed to shape the future of the NHS, or whether the market should be managed to protect the interests of patients and the public. Each point will be considered in turn.

An Emergent Strategy

The reforms which stem from *Working for Patients* are quite unlike previous reorganizations of the NHS in that they are based on a document produced to a tight timetable and which bears all the hallmarks of a strategy only half thought through. There can be no starker contrast than with the 1974 reorganization which derived from a detailed blueprint developed by the Department of Health and Social Security and which, in design at least, left nothing to chance. In effect, managers and professionals have been discovering the importance of the separation of purchaser and provider roles, NHS trusts and GP fundholding and have been developing policy in the course of making the reforms work. Whether this is described as an emergent strategy or 'making it up as we go along', the effect is the same: much of the detail involved in the reforms was missing at their inception and policy has been made on the hoof.

The main benefit of this approach has been to allow those involved in purchasing and providing health services an unusual degree of freedom to influence and shape policy. To a significant extent, the real knowledge about the reforms and the way in which they are working rests with staff in the NHS rather than with civil servants in the Department of Health. This has been associated with a period of almost unprecedented innovation and experimentation in which NHS staff have used the freedoms available to them to test out what the reforms mean in practice. As a consequence, traditional relationships have been turned on their head with those at the centre struggling to keep pace with their colleagues on the ground.

The principal disadvantage of an emergent strategy has been a degree of ambiguity and inconsistency on the part of politicians responsible for the reforms. To oversimplify only a little, the Prime Ministers and Secretaries of State who have been associated with the reforms have each brought his or her agenda to the table (*see* Box 6). In the case of Margaret Thatcher, this was a belief in the value of the market as a means of improving performance. Kenneth Clarke shared this belief and in addition he was concerned to reform primary care through both GP fundholding and the new contract for GPs introduced in 1990. William Waldegrave placed less emphasis on the market during his tenure as Secretary of State and instead gave priority to developing the role of health authorities as planners and purchasers. It was at this stage that the green paper on *The Health of the Nation* was published. Throughout this period Waldegrave stressed the contribution that health authorities could make to delivering the improvements in health set out in the green paper.

John Major, who took over as Prime Minister from Margaret Thatcher in November 1990, added a further layer of policy with the *Citizen's Charter* and its offspring, the *Patient's Charter*. These documents were an attempt to distinguish Majorism from Thatcherism and served to highlight those aspects of the NHS reforms concerned to improve the quality of services from the patient's perspective. To complete the process - at least for the time being -Virginia Bottomley brought a particular interest in community care to the Department of Health and took a number of initiatives in this area, while continuing to oversee the implementation of policies initiated by her predecessors.

Box 6: Changing political priorities.

Margaret Thatcher	Competition and markets
Kenneth Clarke	The reform of primary care
William Waldegrave	*The Health of the Nation*
John Major	*The Patient's Charter*
Virginia Bottomley	Community care

In these circumstances, it would have been surprising if the intentions of the architects of the reforms had not been diluted and to some extent distorted in the implementation process. It could be argued that civil servants provided the continuity that was lacking among politicians but in this respect too there were frequent changes in personnel at a senior level. In addition, there was not always a consistent view on the part of civil servants, particularly as the management executive endeavoured to strengthen its role and the policy divisions in the Department of Health came under challenge. On some issues, such as the Functions and Manpower Review conducted during 1993 (*see* below), former Secretaries of State were able to influence the direction of the reforms through Cabinet-level discussions, but for the most part it was left to the Secretary of State in office, advised by her officials, to place the appropriate interpretation on the intentions of her predecessors. Given that these intentions were expressed in often vague and general terms, and *Working for Patients* itself was a broad framework rather than a detailed blueprint, it was to be expected that policy would be moulded on the basis not only of experience but also personal preferences and political judgement.

The other consequence of an emergent strategy was that difficulties arose during the course of implementation because insufficient thought had been given at the design stage to how the reforms would work in practice. In view of the inability to predict every contingency in advance, this was hardly surprising. Nevertheless, there were occasions when a little more forward planning might have prevented problems occurring. One obvious example concerned the process of setting budgets for GP fundholders. The inequity of a capitation formula for health authorities and an activity-based formula for fundholders quickly became apparent, and it was not easy to see how this could be rectified after the policy had been implemented.

Partly in anticipation of these kinds of problems, the management executive took a close interest in how the reforms were implemented. This first became evident during the course of 1990 when the Chief Executive and Deputy Chief Executive of the NHS indicated that the reforms should be taken forward in a planned and orderly fashion. This was variously described as a smooth take off, steady state and no surprises, but the intent was unambiguous: Ministers and officials wanted to ensure that the new market in health care was introduced slowly and with as little turbulence as possible. Put slightly differently, the aim was to manage the market in the initial stages in order to avoid harmful instability. As time went on, this emerged as a key theme within the reforms as a whole and one that was to test political judgement to its limits.

A Managed Market

The steady state policy was motivated by both political and managerial considerations. On the one hand, Ministers wanted to avoid the NHS reappearing in newspaper headlines in the run up to a general election. The prospect of hospitals finding themselves in financial difficulty as a result of the operation of the market was not attractive to the government and for this reason there was a strong political imperative to ensure that the reforms were implemented smoothly.

On the other hand, managers were aware of the huge programme of change involved in the reforms. Implementing this programme was made easier by the plan to phase in the reforms over a period of years but there was still a great deal to be done to put the basic building blocks in place from April 1991. Those on the inside of this process may one day publish their version of events, but from the outside there was a strong suggestion that both politicians and officials were having second thoughts and were on the verge of aborting take off altogether.

In the event, this did not happen and implementation proceeded under the close eye of the NHS management executive. The *NHS and Community Care Bill* received the Royal Assent at the end of June 1990 paving the way for work to begin in earnest on detailed planning for April 1991. In anticipation of this, the NHS management executive requested health authorities to undertake a stock take of their plans for placing contracts. Health authorities were also advised to concentrate on block contracts to begin with to reduce the level of uncertainty and complexity for providers. In submitting reports to the management executive, health authorities were asked to identify large variations in how services were provided and how they planned to manage the risk of hospitals that depended heavily on income from extra contractual referrals (Ham, 1991).

The concerns of Ministers and civil servants were highlighted by a Department of Health memorandum on the likely effects of the reforms in London that was leaked to the Labour Party during 1990. The memorandum identified a strong possibility that health authorities outside London might decide to treat patients locally instead of referring them to teaching hospitals in London, partly because of the lower costs and spare capacity in the shire counties. The memorandum went on to record that GP fundholders might change their referrals in the same way. The effect would be to destabilize hospital provision in London leading to possible closures and cut backs.

The London memorandum was closely linked to the announcement in December 1990 of the allocation of resources to regional health authorities for 1991/92. Instead of redirecting cash on the weighted capitation basis set out in *Working for Patients*, Ministers gave more money than expected to the Thames regions. This provided a safety net to help authorities in London avoid bed closures and cut backs in the first year of the reforms. At the same time, additional resources were set aside to enable health authorities to clear underlying deficits in their budgets, thereby allowing all hospitals to compete from April 1991 on a comparable basis.

The NHS management executive continued to exercise detailed super-vision of the operation of the reforms during 1991. The result was less a market in which a multitude of transactions took place between buyers and sellers than a command and control bureaucracy of the kind that has been dismantled across central and eastern Europe (Ham, 1992c). The central controls served their purpose by ensuring that the reforms were, on the whole, introduced in an orderly way. Despite well publicized prob-lems at the Guy's and Lewisham and Bradford NHS trusts, which announced plans to make 900 staff redundant shortly after the market came into operation, most services continued to be provided in the same way during 1991/92.

It was, however, clear that it would be difficult to sustain this policy on a long term basis. The logic behind the reforms was that competition would act as a stimulus to improve performance, implying acceptance of a degree of instability as the market began to work. Furthermore, while Ministers may have been cautious about the pace of change, many of those working in the NHS were impatient to exercise the freedoms they believed they had been given. In recognition of this, the management executive announced that the second year of reforms would be a year of managed change in which the market would be allowed to come more fully into play.

In practice the impact of competition was felt most strongly in London and the major conurbations. This was in part because several hospitals in close proximity to each other created the conditions for a market to develop, and in part because of the way in which resources were allocat-ed to district health authorities. The introduction of a weighted capita-tion formula at district level benefited health authorities in the shire coun-ties at the expense of those in the inner cities. As a consequence, money moved away from the relatively expensive hospitals in the inner cities to those in surrounding areas with lower costs and greater accessibility. This was exactly what the Department of Health memorandum on London leaked to the Labour Party had predicted, and in October 1991 the gov-ernment set up an inquiry into the future of health services in London led by Professor Sir Bernard Tomlinson.

At the time the inquiry was established, Ministers announced that four successful applications for NHS trust status in London would not go ahead until April 1993 to allow the recommendations of the Tomlinson inquiry to be taken into account. In this way, the signals thrown up by the market were joined with a strategic overview in an attempt to ensure an orderly process of change. Additional funds were also made available to the Thames regions to assist hospitals unable to attract sufficient contracts to balance their books. Outside London these issues were handled less through Tomlinson-style inquiries than by health authority purchasers working with each other and with providers to plan the reduction in hospital capacity that the market made inevitable. Whatever the preferred approach, the outcome was the same: the internal market became a managed market in which competition and planning went hand in hand.

The Tomlinson inquiry reported in October 1992 (*see* Box 7). In brief, it recommended the closure or merger of 10 inner London hospitals and the concentration of medical education and research on fewer sites. In parallel, proposals were put forward for strengthening primary care services at an estimated cost of £140 million. The *Tomlinson Report* provoked a storm of protest and criticism. With the exception of the plan to develop primary health care services, which received widespread support despite doubts about its feasibility, every aspect of Sir Bernard Tomlinson's analysis came under close scrutiny. Those institutions singled out for closure or major change of use mounted campaigns to oppose the inquiry's recommendations, and attention centred in particular on St Bartholomew's Hospital.

For its part, the government published a response to Tomlinson in February 1993, accepting most of the inquiry's analysis while acknowledging that some of the detailed proposals would need to be re-examined (Department of Health, 1993d). To assist in this process, further reviews were set up into the future of six specialist services and the quality of research in London. The Secretary of State also established the London Implementation Group, under the leadership of a former regional health authority chairman and general manager, to take responsibility for overseeing the process of change in London.

The unanswered question was whether change could be properly planned. On the one hand, health authorities were forcing the pace by moving contracts more rapidly than anticipated by Tomlinson and others. This became evident during 1993 when the Camden and Islington Health Authority announced its plans to move a number of services from University College Hospital (UCH) to other hospitals because of price differentials (Brindle, 1993a). On the other hand, GP fundholders did not always agree with the plans and priorities of health authorities and indicated their willingness to use their resources to frustrate these plans.

Box 7: The Tomlinson Report.

The *Tomlinson Report* recommended a shift of focus in London. This included increasing expenditure on primary care and community health services and reducing the number of hospitals and beds. The major changes affecting hospital services in the *Tomlinson Report* were:

- the redevelopment of University College Hospital (UCH) and the Middlesex on the UCH site

- the merger of St Bartholomew's and the Royal London hospitals on the Royal London site

- the merger of Guy's and St Thomas's on one site

- a rationalization of services in west London following the opening of the Westminster-Chelsea Hospital affecting the Charing Cross and Hammersmith hospitals among others

These changes were intended to rationalize the provision of specialist services on fewer sites and reduce the number of beds by between 2,000 and 7,000 by the end of the decade.

Source: Tomlinson Report (1992)

This emerged as a key factor in south west London where Queen Mary's University Hospital in Roehampton was strongly supported by fundholders, even though a review undertaken by health authorities in the area identified it as the hospital most likely to close as services were rationalized from four sites to three (Brindle, 1993b).

The dilemma here for the government was that having deliberately moved away from old style, centralized planning to a more pluralistic set of arrangements, in which greater power was given to purchasers and providers at a local level, it became difficult to direct what happened in the NHS from the centre. In practice, Ministers did intervene in the market, not only to enforce a steady state in the first year but also to ensure that change was planned thereafter. As an example, the Camden and Islington Health Authority was instructed not to move contracts away from UCH in order that the rationalization of hospital services in that part of London went ahead as planned. In acting in this way Ministers were responding (whether consciously or not) to the concern expressed by Sir Bernard Tomlinson a year after publication of his report that the government had not intervened sufficiently in the market and that a more managed approach to change was needed.

41

Yet by intervening, Ministers ran the risk of weakening the imperatives facing providers in a competitive environment to cut their costs and raise standards. While a managed market called for some intervention on the part of Ministers and officials, the danger this gave rise to was the creation of a culture in which providers who were unsuccessful knew that they would receive political protection and extra funding. The result would be the worst of both worlds: a mixture of bureaucratic controls coupled with the additional transaction costs of the market, with the benefits of neither approach.

Striking the right balance between management and the market was crucial to the success of the reforms and yet, as part of the emergent strategy, it was an issue whose significance was only recognized during the course of implementation. Although some work was done behind the scenes by civil servants and NHS managers, it was not until the end of 1993, when Ministers set in hand a series of reviews to define the functions to be performed in the NHS in future, that regulating and managing the market was even acknowledged to be a key issue. In the absence of a clear lead from the centre, it was left to local purchasers and providers to work out their best way forward, often with the support and assistance of regional health authorities and management executive outposts. This resulted in major reviews of the future of hospital and health services in areas such as Birmingham, Bristol, West Yorkshire and Newcastle. What these reviews did not address was how the market would be managed on a continuing basis.

The Impact on Patients

In analysing the impact of the reforms, it is as well to remember the title of the white paper from which they derive. *Working for Patients* may have been a response to financial and managerial problems in the NHS but its ostensible purpose was to improve services to patients. Fascinating as innovations such as GP fundholding and NHS trusts may be, the ultimate test of the reforms is what difference they have made for patients. This is the yardstick against which the success or failure of the reforms should be judged and it is here that the debate continues between the government and its critics.

When Ministers assess the impact of the reforms on patients, they emphasize two factors above all others. First, they claim that more patients are being treated than ever before, citing an increase of 16 per cent in hospital activity levels between 1990 and 1993 in support of this view. Ministers also argue that activity rates have increased more quickly than in the period before the reforms and that NHS trusts have out-performed hospitals that are not yet trusts.

Second, Ministers maintain that there have been improvements in waiting times, especially for those patients waiting a long time for an operation. This is usually attributed to the *Patient's Charter* which, when it was published in 1991, promised that no patients should wait longer than two years for surgery. Beyond these specific claims, Ministers also contend that there has been an overall improvement in quality as NHS trusts have responded to the challenge of the market to raise standards of care. In this case, examples such as improved access to services and initiatives to enhance patient convenience are invoked to illustrate the impact of the reforms.

While there is an element of truth in all of these claims, they need to be treated with caution. To begin with, the increase in the number of patients treated is arguably the result of the additional funding provided for the NHS in recent years rather than the reforms *per se* (Bloor and Maynard, 1993). The rate of growth in NHS spending was significantly greater in the period 1990-93 than during the 1980s and this undoubtedly enabled more patients to be treated (*see* Table 1). There is also anecdotal evidence to suggest that providers have improved their systems for counting and recording the work done. Some of the increase in activity that has occurred is almost certainly an artefact of better information systems rather than a reflection of genuine productivity gains.

The reduction in waiting times should be viewed in a similar light. The longest waiting times have indeed fallen and no patient now has to wait longer than two years for an operation. There has also been a reduction in the number of patients waiting between one and two years. To some extent, however, these improvements have been achieved at the expense of an increase in the number of patients waiting for less than a year. Equally significant is the fact that the reduction in waiting times has been brought about less by the market than through earmarked funding and direct political intervention. Ministers have made it clear that the jobs of health authority chairmen and general managers who fail to deliver the government's targets are on the line, and it is this that has served as a spur to improved performance.

As far as overall improvements in quality are concerned, it is difficult to sustain the argument that the reforms have been responsible for any

Table 1: Net UK NHS spending.

Year (£M)	HCHS (5)	FHS (6)	Capital	Total cash (1)	Total real (3)	Cash index	Inflation index	% Real change
1983/4 (2)	10767	3412	896	15553	15553	100.0	100.0	–
1984/5 (2)	11398	3747	984	16673	16783	107.2	106.5	0.7
1985/6 (2)	12018	3966	1048	17633	17843	113.4	112.0	0.5
1986/7	13250	3848	1153	18860	19203	121.3	119.1	0.6
1987/8	14605	4272	1135	20700	21439	133.1	128.5	1.7
1988/9	16213	4814	1145	22892	23793	147.2	141.6	0.4
1989/90	17382	5017	1514	24724	26158	159.0	150.3	1.8
1990/1	19471	5574	1731	27699	30260	178.1	163.0	3.3
1991/2	22471	6209	1657	31420	35364	202.0	179.5	3.0
1992/3 (est outturn)	24859	6547	1915	34564	39626 (4)	222.2	193.8	1.9

Source: The Government's Expenditure Plans: 1993/4 to 1995/6

Notes:
1. Total includes: central health and misc. services and Department Administration
2. Figures for HCHS and FHS before 1986/7 not comparable with later years
3. Total spending at constant prices using NHS pay and prices index as deflator
4. Deflated figures using Health Services Management Centre estimates of NHS inflation
5. Hospital and community health services
6. Family health services

dramatic change of policy or practice. Raising the standard of health care has been an issue high on the health policy agenda right through the 1980s and was emphasized particularly in the *Griffiths Report* of 1983. As a consequence, there have been many improvements in service provision and a stronger focus on the patient's perspective. The nature of the changes that have occurred has been demonstrated in a series of reports and studies. The NHS reforms may have helped to continue what was already happening and given fresh impetus to existing initiatives but they did not in any sense represent a radical departure from previous policies to improve quality.

So what has been the impact of the reforms on patients? The most important effect has been to change the balance of power within the NHS (Ham, 1993a), illustrated in the Figures 4-7. Whereas in the past, the NHS was organized along two parallel tracks which rarely came into contact, this is no longer the case.

Figure 4: The old NHS

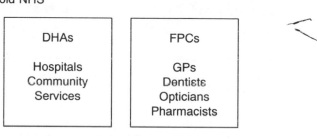

DHAs	FPCs
Hospitals	GPs
Community	Dentists
Services	Opticians
	Pharmacists

Figure 5: The purchaser/provider split.

DHAs as purchasers	FHSAs
NHS Trusts	GPs
Hospitals	Dentists
Community	Opticians
Services	Pharmacists

Purchaser and provider roles have been separated, district health authorities have opened up a dialogue with GPs, and the developing alliance between district health authorities and GPs has put pressure on providers to improve their performance. Add to this the stimulus offered by GP fundholding, and the effect has been to enhance the accountability of providers to purchasers and to open up a debate about the standards of care that should be delivered.

Figure 6: DHAs form alliances with GPs.

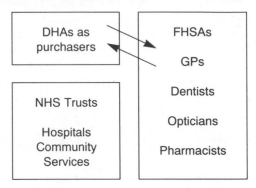

Figure 7: DHA/GP alliances put pressure on providers.

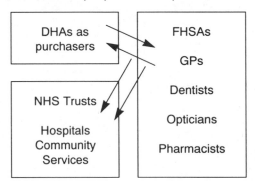

The old system of planning by decibels, in which the providers of acute services won the biggest share of resources, has been brought into question, and there has been a shift of emphasis in favour of primary care. It follows that GPs occupy a pivotal position in the new NHS with resources and services moving increasingly in the direction of primary care. To this extent, the agenda promoted by Kenneth Clarke rather than Margaret Thatcher (see above) has come to prevail. Four examples illustrate these developments.

First, there is increasing emphasis on the development of shared care between GPs and specialists in areas such as asthma and diabetes. Second, specialists in some districts are holding their out-patient clinics in GPs' surgeries rather than in hospitals. This often involves 'treat and teach' arrangements in which GPs develop their own skills by sitting in on the consultation. Third, many practices are carrying out a wider range of diagnostic tests in their surgeries, thereby reducing demands on hospitals. And fourth, GPs are employing additional staff in primary care teams to enable them to deliver more services to patients, for example, physiotherapists, chiropodists, dietitians and counsellors.

Taken together, these developments are profoundly altering the shape of the NHS. In organizational terms, the old hierarchical, integrated structures have been replaced by a more diverse (some would say fragmented) set of contractual arrangements. Within these arrangements, established relationships have come into question. The stronger focus on primary care developed by GPs, health authorities and fundholders has been matched by rapid changes in relation to secondary care and considerable uncertainty as to the future pattern of hospital services. Hospital managers and professionals have found their own position under increasing challenge as those involved in primary care have come to exert greater influence.

Nowhere is this better illustrated than in relation to GP fundholding. With the purchasing power to back their decisions, fundholders are in a strong position to negotiate improvements in services on behalf of their patients. This they have done in a range of ways, including offering additional services in their practices, cutting waiting times for out-patient appointments and elective surgery, and improving communication with hospital doctors and managers. Ministers have used these changes in support of the argument that the reforms really are working for patients. Despite this, doubts continue to be expressed about the impact of fundholding in the longer term.

The critics of fundholding marshalled several arguments to question the viability of the scheme (summarized in Ham, 1992e). To begin with they contend that only large, well managed practices have been involved in the scheme so far. As the experience of these practices was unlikely to be typical of GPs as a whole, it was not possible to generalize from the early evidence on fundholding and seek to judge its success in the longer term. Not least, given the support received by fundholders in the first and second waves, in order to get the scheme off the ground, the risks involved had been minimized but were likely to become more apparent with time.

Foremost among these risks is the incentive for GPs to be more careful in their selection of patients. This did not emerge as a problem in the initial stages of fundholding because GPs received a budget which reflected fully the use their patients made of services in the past. However, reports indicated that some fundholders were resisting the acceptance of high-cost patients during 1993 (Timmins, 1993). The planned move to a weighted capitation formula for fundholders increased the likelihood of this happening, if the formula was not sufficiently sophisticated to allow fully for the cost of treating patients with different medical histories and clinical conditions.

A related risk was that GPs would have an incentive to underrefer patients to hospitals. The argument here was that with financial as well as clinical factors entering into the decision on when to seek a specialist opinion, GPs might choose to make fewer referrals in order to keep within budgets or to make savings. If this were to happen, it would undermine trust between patients and their doctors, particularly as patients became more aware of the way in which fundholding operated.

The danger of underreferral was accentuated by the arrangement under which fundholders paid for elective care but not emergency treatment; if a GP waited until a patient's condition warranted emergency admission the bill for treatment would fall to the health authority. A significant increase in emergency admissions experienced by hospitals in many parts of the NHS during 1993 gave rise to the suspicion that this factor was beginning to come into play, although there was no evidence that fundholding was more important than other influences in accounting for this rise.

A further risk was that standards within general practice would widen as a result of fundholding. Put another way, good primary care services would become even better as GPs in well run practices took advantage of fundholding to improve their services to patients. This would do little to assist smaller practices, particularly single handed GPs working from inadequate premises in deprived inner city districts. As such, fundholding would accentuate the inverse care law, a risk that was highlighted by the concentration of fundholding in the early stages in those areas where standards of care were already high. By contrast, fundholders were few and far between in the inner cities.

These and other factors stimulated a lively debate both within the NHS and among academic observers. The latter were divided in their attempts to evaluate the impact of fundholding. Glennerster and his colleagues reached a conclusion that was generally positive (Glennerster and others, 1992), whereas other observers were more cautious. Coulter, for example, argued that:

'fundholding remains an interesting experiment . . . but we have not arrived at the point where general practitioners should take over as the main purchasers of health care' (Coulter, 1992, p397).

As a number of observers pointed out, alongside the benefits of fundholding had to be set the costs. With a preparatory fee of £16,000, an annual management allowance of £34,000, a significant investment in computers and information systems, and the additional effort required of providers in negotiating tailor-made contracts with an expanding number of small purchasers, fundholding was an expensive way of organising the purchasing function. It also placed a significant management responsibility on GPs and this emerged as the main drawback perceived by those involved in fundholding.

Partly in response to this, there was increasing interest in the establishment of fundholding consortia. These consortia, often referred to as multifunds or superfunds, involved collaboration between fundholders in several practices. The aim was to achieve the benefits of fundholding while reducing the management effort involved. Fundholding consortia typically employed a number of managers to act on behalf of the participating practices, although responsibility for managing the fund remained at the practice level. The formation of consortia resulted in greater convergence between fundholding and district health authority purchasing, particularly as district health authorities used a variety of means to involve GPs in their purchasing decisions. In both cases, the aim was to combine the sensitivity of a patient-centred approach to purchasing with the leverage and economies of scale of a population-centred approach.

Managing the New NHS

The concern over management costs was not confined to fundholding. During the course of 1993, through a series of Parliamentary questions, Alan Milburn, a backbench Labour MP, extracted information from the Department of Health on the increase in the number of managers that had resulted from the reforms. This illustrated that in the UK the number of managers rose from 6,091 in 1989/90 to 20,478 in 1992/93. Over the same period the number of administrative and clerical staff rose from 144,582 to 166,363. There was a much smaller increase in the numbers of other staff employed in the NHS.

While some of the increase in management costs could be explained by a reclassification of nursing staff into management grades, there was also a real growth in the number of managers employed as a direct result of government policies. Part of this cost increase arose from the 1983 Griffiths' reforms and the remainder was due to the extra workload following *Working for Patients*. It became clear that the shift from an integrated to a contract system involved additional transaction costs associated with negotiating and monitoring contracts and related billing and invoicing arrangements. What was difficult to judge was whether the expenditure on management had produced commensurate benefits in terms of gains in efficiency and improvements in quality.

Prompted by concerns about the increase in management costs, the Secretary of State for Wales, John Redwood, placed a moratorium on new management posts in Wales and issued guidance asking health authorities and trusts to reduce the percentage of their budgets spent on management. In a thinly veiled attack on the policies of his predecessors, Redwood criticized the number of 'men in grey suits' in the NHS and called for a reduction in bureaucracy to enable more money to be spent on direct patient care. As this debate developed, the Functions and Manpower Review, initiated by Virginia Bottomley, was examining how the structure of the NHS should be changed to bring it into line with the objectives of the reforms.

The Functions and Manpower Review grew out of an analysis of the intermediate tier of management begun in 1992 (Ham, 1993b). This analysis focused particularly on the respective roles of regional health authorities and management executive outposts, and their relationship with purchasers and providers. At the beginning of 1993 the Secretary of State announced that regional health authorities had been asked to reduce the number of staff they employed to a maximum of 200 each. At the same time, she established the Functions and Manpower Review under the leadership of Kate Jenkins, from the NHS Policy Board, and Alan Langlands, Deputy Chief Executive of the NHS.

The terms of reference eventually agreed for the Review were wide ranging, encompassing not only the role of the intermediate tier but also the work of the Department of Health as well as management arrangements at a local level. The Jenkins/Langlands Review reported to the Secretary of State in July 1993 setting out various options for consideration. The government's decisions on these options were announced in October 1993 in a report entitled *Managing the New NHS* (Ham, 1993c). These decisions centred on three key elements: the merger of district health authorities and family health services authorities; the abolition of regional health authorities; and a streamlined NHS management executive operating through eight regional offices. Cutting across all these elements was a policy of reducing management costs.

In one sense, these proposals were a tidying up exercise designed to reduce duplication and clarify management arrangements. This was behind the decision to abolish regional health authorities and to merge district health authorities and family health services authorities. Similarly, the changes to the management executive were intended to reduce central intervention in the NHS and establish the management executive clearly as the head office of the NHS within the Department of Health. The creation of regional offices of the management executive also meant that for the first time there would be a single agency at the regional level in a position to relate to both purchasers and providers. It also opened up the possibility that regional offices, acting as part of the civil service rather than the NHS, would strengthen rather than weaken central control of health services.

More fundamentally, the outcome of the Functions and Manpower Review can be seen as an attempt to address the question of where to strike a balance between management and competition. By abolishing regional health authorities and streamlining the management executive, the government opened up the possibility of the market developing more rapidly, free of bureaucratic intervention. This was certainly the aspiration of Kenneth Clarke who maintained a close interest in the Review. In practice, much will depend on how the new regional offices of the management executive take on their role and the way in which they are used by their political masters. The fact that a regional structure has been retained at all, when some were arguing for its complete abolition, suggests that Ministers recognize the dangers of unrestricted competition and are committed to regulating the operation of the market. But precisely how this will be done remains to be seen.

A number of the changes contained in *Managing the New NHS* cannot be introduced without legislation. This applies particularly to the abolition of regional health authorities and the merger of district health authorities and family health services authorities. The government has announced that a bill will be introduced into Parliament in the 1994/95 session and if approved will come into effect from April 1996. In the meantime, the number of regional health authorities was reduced from 14

Figure 8: New structure of the NHS.

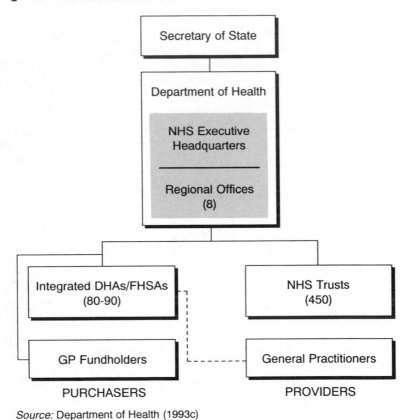

Source: Department of Health (1993c)

to eight and plans are proceeding to reorganize the work of the NHS executive (the new title of the managed executive). Subject to legislation, the new structure of the NHS will emerge as in Figure 8.

Managing the New NHS was similar to *Working for Patients* in that it indicated the overall direction of the government's thinking without the supporting detail. Accordingly, 12 functions' analysis groups were

Figure 9: Functions carried out by the NHS.

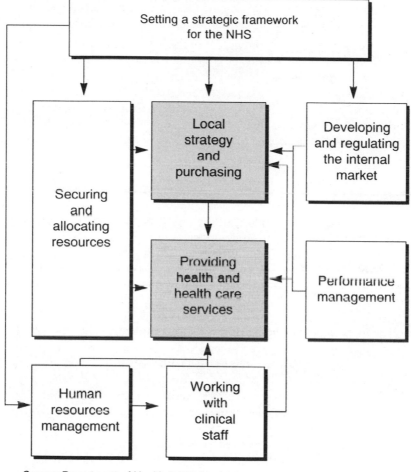

Source: Department of Health (1993c)

53

established to supply this detail. These groups focused on the eight key areas identified in *Managing the New NHS* (*see* Figure 9). In addition, groups were set up to look at estates' management, information, communications and cross functional issues.

Taken together, these decisions amounted to nothing less than a further reorganization of the NHS, perhaps not on the scale of *Working for Patients*, but in some ways equally significant. Echoing the starting point of this chapter, this reorganization was necessary because, in the spirit of an emergent strategy, it had become clear that the structure of the NHS was no longer in tune with the requirements of the reforms. In this case, a Secretary of State who was intuitively unsympathetic to structural change, was persuaded of the need to take action, both because of the logic of developments within the NHS and because of wider developments within government. As far as the latter was concerned, the pressures on government spending and the need to search for savings at every opportunity meant that NHS management costs could not be exempt from scrutiny. Both the Prime Minister's Office and the Treasury were involved in the Functions and Manpower Review and pressure from these sources helped to force the pace of change.

Conclusion

In this chapter, we have analysed the impact of the reforms in the first three years of operation. In so doing we have highlighted the evolutionary nature of the reforms and the increasing understanding that has been gained of their impact during the process of implementation. It has become clear that a delicate balance has to be struck between management and competition and Ministers have demonstrated their willingness to intervene in the market when required so to do.

The most important effect of the reforms to date has been to change the balance of power within the NHS. This has made providers more accountable to purchasers and it has strengthened the position of primary care. GP fundholding has been at the forefront of these developments, although doubts remain about the long term viability of the fundholding scheme. As a consequence of these changes, there has been a fundamental shift in views and attitudes within the NHS and an ability to tackle problems that previously appeared intractable.

One of the concerns that has emerged is the increase in management costs that has resulted from the reforms. This applies throughout the

NHS and was a key factor behind the Functions and Manpower Review conducted during 1993. As a result of the Review, the NHS is in the throes of a further reorganization. This will have the effect of changing the structure of the NHS yet again as well as seeking to reduce management costs.

The impact of the reforms on patients is more difficult to assess. The claims made by Ministers of increases in the number of patients treated and reductions in waiting times need to be treated cautiously. Insofar as there have been improvements in these areas, they are probably the consequence of increased levels of funding for the NHS in the period since 1990 rather than the reforms alone. More positively, patients in some parts of the NHS have benefited from the changes to primary care that have occurred, although there are continuing concerns about morale in general practice (see below). A proper judgement about the impact of the reforms needs to be made over a longer period of time on the basis of a wider range of evidence. To this extent, the jury is still out.

The Future of the NHS Reforms

At the time of writing, the Major government is in the midst of a fundamental review of public expenditure designed to ask searching questions about all aspects of public spending. The review was stimulated by a public sector borrowing requirement of £50 billion in 1993/94 and by the need to assess whether current spending plans can be sustained into the next century. During 1993 the review focused particularly on social security, including expenditure on state pensions, child benefit and invalidity benefit. Towards the end of that year press reports indicated that attention was turning to the NHS with suggestions that charges might be introduced to cover some of the costs of patients staying in hospital as a way of generating additional resources. This raised the prospect that the future of the NHS might again be placed under the microscope with the more radical options that were discarded during the 1988 Ministerial Review coming back onto the table.

International Experience

The government's review of public expenditure is taking place against a background of health care reform in many countries. As a variety of studies have shown, there are a number of common themes in health care reform (Ham, Robinson and Benzeval, 1990; OECD, 1992). In the 1970s and early 1980s the principal objective was to contain the growth of health services expenditure. This was achieved in all countries with the exception of the United States, through a mixture of global budgets for hospitals, controls over doctors' fees and incomes, and limitations on the building of new hospitals and the acquisition of medical technology.

In the latter half of the 1980s the focus shifted to ways of achieving greater efficiency in the use of resources, increasing patient choice and improving the quality of care. These policies were pursued using a variety of instruments. First, priority was given to strengthening the management of health services. This included moving from a tradition of administration to a culture of management, seeking to involve clinicians in management, and exploring ways of managing clinical activity more effectively. The initiatives taken in this area encompassed medical audit and peer review, the use of managed care arrangements, and an emphasis on technology assessment and health services accreditation.

Second, there was increasing interest in the development of budgetary incentives. While global budgets for hospitals and caps on doctors' fees were largely successful in containing overall levels of expenditure, they were much less effective in promoting efficiency in the use of resources at the micro level. In response, policy makers sought to combine controls on total spending with incentives for both doctors and hospitals. This included altering the fee schedule for doctors, making use of capitation payments, and experimenting with the use of cost per case payments for hospitals, such as diagnosis related groups.

Third, of growing importance in health care reform was the use of markets as well as management as a stimulus to efficiency and responsiveness. In no case did this involve abandoning management in the pursuit of free market solutions. Rather, it meant searching for the middle ground in the belief that this would provide a more effective way of improving the performance of health services than the established approaches (see Figure 10). Thus, just as market oriented systems showed greater interest in management, so managed systems began testing out competitive approaches. To this extent there was a convergence around managed competition as a strategy for reform, although it should be emphasized that managed competition meant different things in different places.

Figure 10: Trends in health care reforms.

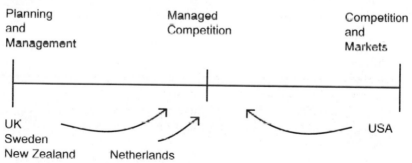

A fourth theme came on to the agenda in the first half of the 1990s as a number of countries initiated reviews of the scope of their health services. Of particular relevance to the United Kingdom was the work done in The Netherlands and New Zealand (Ministry of Welfare, Health and

Cultural Affairs, 1992; National Advisory Committee, 1992). In both countries, government-appointed committees were set up to advise on the basic benefits' packages (in The Netherlands) or core services (in New Zealand) to be covered in the publicly-funded health services. As the work of these committees demonstrated, it was not easy to draw a clear distinction between services in the core and those outside. Choices in health care involved a complex set of judgements and it was necessary to draw on scientific evidence, professional advice and public values in determining priorities. This was underscored by experience in Oregon where the initiative taken by the state government to set priorities for the Medicaid System attracted widespread interest.

Underlying these themes in health care reform were a number of more fundamental issues. To begin with, it was clear that all systems faced similar problems, almost regardless of the methods and levels of funding. These problems included evidence of inefficiency in the use of resources, poor integration between secondary care, primary care and social care, an over emphasis on hospital services, and the relative neglect of primary care (Ham, Robinson and Benzeval, 1990). In view of this, it is not surprising that reform has focused more on the delivery of services than their financing.

Following on from this, it is also apparent that there are no quick-fix solutions to the problems faced by the health care systems of developed countries. In almost all countries there is dissatisfaction with the effectiveness of existing policies and a search for new policy instruments. In this context, policy makers have shown increasing interest in the experience of health care systems other than their own in the hope that this may hold some pointers to the future.

This helps to explain the degree of convergence in health care reform in different countries. It also accounts for the extent of interest in the United Kingdom experience, where the process of reform has gone ahead more rapidly than in many other countries. In this respect, the NHS has become a laboratory for the rest of the world, particularly in illustrating what happens when a market is grafted on to a publicly financed and managed health service (Ham, 1993d).

To argue that there are no quick-fix solutions to the problems faced by health policy makers is to urge caution in the pursuit of radical alternatives. In the context of the fundamental review of public expenditure taking place in the United Kingdom, it suggests that the lesson of the 1980s should not be forgotten. On two occasions Margaret Thatcher's governments considered and rejected changing the basis of financing health services by moving towards a system of private or social insurance, with the opportunity for citizens to opt out into a private insurance scheme. There seems no reason to alter this judgement, even though there are those who continue to argue in favour of such an approach. As Nigel Lawson notes in his memoirs:

> 'we looked . . . at other countries to see whether we could learn from them; but it was soon clear that every country we looked at was having problems with its provision of medical care. All of them – France, the United States, Germany – had different systems; but each of them had acute problems which none of them had solved. They were all in at least as much difficulty as we were, and it did not take long to conclude that there was surprisingly little that we could learn from any of the other systems. To try to change from the Health Service to any of the sorts of systems in use overseas would simply be out of the frying pan into the fire' (Lawson, 1992, p616).

If this is accepted, then a more promising way forward is to build on the implementation of the *Working for Patients* reforms and to strengthen these reforms in the light of the experience gained since 1991. The fact that countries as diverse as The Netherlands, New Zealand and Sweden are pursuing similar reforms (*see* Box 8) reinforces this conclusion. With the experience of three years of the NHS reforms on which to draw, it is possible to identify some tentative lessons and to suggest what needs to be done to take the reforms forward. In so doing, it is also possible to suggest how a future Labour government might adapt the reforms in pursuing its objectives.

Market Management

As the reforms move into their next phase, the major challenge continues to be to achieve a balance between the stimulus of the market and the need for the market to be managed. The underlying rationale for market management is that competition may run counter to the principles and values of a publicly funded health care system. Safeguards therefore are needed to protect the principles on which the NHS is based and to prevent behaviour which is anti-competitive. In earlier chapters we argued that the nature of market management has been neglected by Ministers and their advisors. This needs to be rectified as a matter of urgency, as competition plays a bigger part in shaping the future pattern of service provision.

The essential elements of market management are illustrated in the accompanying box (*see* also Ham and Maynard, 1994). As a starting point, there must be openness of information and a common vocabulary

Box 8: International experience of health care reform.

In **The Netherlands** the Dekker Report of 1987 made proposals for reforming the Dutch health care system designed to introduce competition between providers and insurers. This was to be achieved by insurers offering a basic insurance package paid for partly through payroll contributions and partly through a nominal premium. The size of the premium varies between insurers and this is intended over time to stimulate competition between insurers. In turn, insurers will contract selectively with providers (both doctors and hospitals). Dekker argued that selective contracting would create competition among providers and would thereby result in greater efficiency. The Dekker reforms have been amended in the 'Plan-Simons' and are being implemented gradually over a period of many years. In parallel, the government set up a review of health care priorities and the report, *Choices in Health Care*, was published in 1992.

Health care reform in **Sweden** is proceeding at both a national and local level. A number of county councils have launched experiments with internal markets, the most advanced examples being those in Bohus, Dalarna and Stockholm. These involve a separation of purchaser and provider roles, the use of performance related reimbursement, and a degree of competition among providers. At a national level, the government has appointed two committees to review the financing and organization of health services, and rationing and priority setting. The committee on organization and financing reported in 1993 and described three models of reform. These were an insurance based model, a reformed county council model building on the local initiatives already taking place, and a primary care model involving GP fundholding. The government is expected to announce its decisions during 1994.

Like Sweden and The Netherlands, **New Zealand** is reviewing both the financing and organization of health services, and health care priorities. 14 area health boards have been replaced by four regional health authorities. These regional authorities act as purchasing agencies, buying services from a range of hospitals. Public providers operate as crown health enterprises and compete for contracts from purchasers. In parallel, a government-appointed Core Services Committee has been reviewing the scope of health service provision.

for contracting purposes enabling purchasers to compare providers on a consistent basis. When purchasers and providers cannot agree, an independent, third party is needed to arbitrate in disputes and act as an honest broker. There should also be an agreed set of rules for handling mergers and takeovers.

An important aspect of market management is the ability to oversee the interaction of purchasers and providers and to spot gaps in service provision when they occur. The obverse is the need to avoid unnecessary duplication of services. In some cases purchasers will choose not to give priority to innovations in service provision which are desirable when seen from the perspective of the NHS as a whole. There must be the capacity to fund these innovations in future. Equally, as experience in London and other areas has shown, market management entails the development of exit strategies for coping with providers who compete unsuccessfully in the NHS market.

A further function is to ensure that core values, such as equity and access, are not sacrificed as competition grows in importance. This issue has significance well beyond a discussion of market management as it lies at the heart of current efforts to reform health services. Policy makers are

Box 9: Market management functions in the NHS.

To ensure openness of information and a common vocabulary for contracting purposes

To arbitrate in disputes between purchasers and providers and to act as an honest broker

To oversee mergers and takeovers between purchasers and providers

To supervise the interaction of purchasers and providers and to spot gaps in service provision when they occur

To ensure that there is funding for innovation in service provision that cannot be funded by purchasers

To develop exit strategies for coping with providers who compete unsuccessfully

To ensure that core values such as equity and access are not sacrificed as competition grows in importance continually weighing the trade-offs that should be made between values such as equity, access, efficiency and responsiveness, and it would be wrong to reduce these judgements to technical matters located at an appropriate point in the management structure. Nevertheless, on a day to day basis the priorities of politicians have to be interpreted by civil servants and health service managers and a way of carrying out this function in the NHS has to be found.

Responsibility for undertaking market management rests at several levels. To begin with, district health authorities have a role to play, acting either singly or in combination. They have already demonstrated their ability to act in this way in many parts of the country by taking the initiative to review the pattern of service provision and this function will assume even greater importance in future.

The NHS executive also has a contribution to make. The rules which govern the operation of the market are best set nationally to ensure a level playing field in all parts of the NHS. These rules concern transparency and consistency of information, policies on mergers and takeovers, arbitration procedures, the protection of core values and exit strategies. Their administration is best undertaken by the new regional offices of the NHS executive who for the first time are in a position to relate to both purchasers and providers. This is preferable to the formation of a separate regulatory agency of the kind that exists in the former public utilities such as gas, electricity and water. The NHS presents a different set of challenges to these industries, not least in the strong political influence exerted over the purchasing and provision of health care. For this reason, market management cannot be delegated to an independent regulatory agency but should remain firmly within the structure of the NHS.

Contestability

The future of market management is closely related to the type of competition that will develop within the NHS. An important distinction to be drawn here is between competitive tendering and contestability. A policy of competitive tendering for clinical services would involve purchasers seeking tenders from competing providers for their contracts on a regular basis. This is the policy that has been pursued in relation to support services such as laundry, catering and cleaning, and it is also being used in some areas of clinical care.

In contrast, contestability entails not a formal and regular tendering process but rather the ability of purchasers to switch contracts between providers if they are unable to achieve improvements in performance through other mechanisms. In this case, it is the *threat* of contracts being moved that stimulates providers to respond to the demands of purchasers rather than the reality of moving contracts. Of course, for the threat to be credible purchasers must be prepared to change providers from time to time, but it is the psychology of competition that matters more than its exercise.

Applying these ideas to clinical services in the NHS, it can be argued that contestability would be a more appropriate policy to pursue in most cases than competitive tendering. There are a number of reasons for this. One important factor is the high costs associated with entry and exit in to the health care market. In a publicly funded service, these costs are born by the tax payer and the efficiency gains to result from competitive tendering are unlikely to be sufficient to outweigh the transitional costs involved.

Another factor is experience of purchaser/provider relationships outside the health sector. Evidence from a number of industries indicates that the most effective relationships are those where purchasers and providers work together in long term, collaborative arrangements rather than relationships in which purchasers seek continual short term gains by switching contracts between providers. In the health sector, this approach finds expression in the notion of 'preferred providers', that is, providers who are preferred by purchasers or insurers because they meet certain requirements.

A further consideration is that the scope for competition varies enormously within the NHS. While the market has been quick to develop in London and the major conurbations, it has been much less in evidence in other areas. The reality in many parts of the NHS is of a substantial purchaser faced with a substantial provider and with little alternative but to contract with that provider for many services.

To argue the merits of contestability is not to rule out the use of competitive tendering in some cases. If there are compelling reasons to open up the provision of services to this kind of approach, such as the failure of an existing provider to improve performance after repeated efforts so to do, then this option should be pursued in areas where competing providers exist. But for most services most of the time, a commitment on the part of purchasers and providers to work together in partnership to increase efficiency and raise standards is likely to be more appropriate.

This is not the same as a return to the integration of purchasers and providers within district health authorities. Rather it is to recognize the value of a clear and complete separation of purchaser and provider roles coupled with the ability of purchasers to place contracts with the provider of their choice and not simply those that they manage directly. In this arrangement, the point of separating purchaser and provider roles is less to stimulate a competitive market in health care than to promote greater accountability on the part of providers through the vehicle of contracts (Ham, 1990c). To be sure, competition has a contribution to make to this process but it is merely one of the weapons available to purchasers rather than the principle on which the delivery of services is based.

Seen in this light, contestability depends on purchasers and providers recognizing their common interest in collaborating to improve performance and employing a range of management tools to ensure that this happens. This includes making use of indicators of performance drawn from providers in comparable circumstances. It was this philosophy that underpinned William Waldegrave's attitude to the NHS reforms. As he explained in an interview, the internal market:

> 'isn't a market in the real sense . . . it's competition in the sense that there will be comparative information available. It's not a market in that people don't go bust and make profits and all that, but it's using market-like mechanisms to provide better information' (Smith, 1991, p712).

In this approach, which is sometimes referred to as yardstick competition, the presumption is that behaviour will change in response to information and management intervention as well as through competition. Furthermore, because the emphasis is on partnership relationships, there is less need for the costly monitoring systems, which are an inherent element of contracting relationships in which purchasers and providers are not familiar with each other. In this context the United States' experience is instructive, indicating as it does that insurers and providers in the American system are developing closer working relationships to avoid incurring these costs.

Incentives

One of the major weaknesses of the NHS reforms to date has been the failure to devise adequate budgetary incentives to overcome the efficiency trap faced by providers and which gave rise to the reforms in the first place. A system in which money follows the patient appeared to provide the solution to this problem but in practice, as we have noted, money is not yet following patients in most parts of the NHS. Although purchasers have started to draw up more sophisticated contracts, including the use of rewards and penalties, there is a long way to go before providers are appropriately compensated for improved performance.

The dilemma here is that budgetary incentives are known to have a powerful effect on behaviour in the health services (Eisenberg, 1986). This is well illustrated by the new contract for GPs introduced in 1990. Family doctors responded to the extra payments included in the contract by increasing the range of health promotion work carried out in general practice and achieving higher rates of coverage for vaccination, immunization and cervical cancer screening. The consequence of these and other changes was that GPs were each paid on average £6,000 more in the first year than the government had estimated. In one respect this could be interpreted as a success, but in another respect it was a problem for a government seeking to control the growth of expenditure. Questions were also raised about the cost effectiveness of the services GPs were paid to provide.

A similar lesson emerges from an internal market experiment which has been running in Stockholm since 1992. In many ways this sought to emulate the NHS reforms, except that hospitals were paid for each patient treated in a cost per case system based on diagnosis related groups. Anticipating that activity levels would increase, Stockholm County Council reduced the prices that hospitals charged by 10 per cent in 1992 compared with 1991. Despite this, the number of patients treated increased by considerably more than 10 per cent and while this had a beneficial effect on waiting times it caused financial difficulties for purchasers who were operating with cash limited budgets.

If greater use is made of budgetary incentives within the NHS, a way will have to be found of avoiding these difficulties. And to return to an earlier point, this is exactly the challenge thrown down by GP fundholding. As the financial constraints under which fundholders operate begin to bite, there is a risk that GPs will keep within their budgets by discriminating against patients who are older and sicker and by reducing referrals. To deny this risk is to fly in the face of the wide range of evidence that exists about the impact of budgetary incentives on clinical practice patterns, including evidence that fundholders themselves have increased expenditure on drugs at a slower rate than non-fundholders. It is of course open to GPs to opt out of fundholding or indeed to refuse to stay within budgets. The latter position is however tenable only on a short term basis as it will quickly lead to the withdrawal of fundholding status for the practices concerned.

The point behind these examples is that budgetary incentives are not only powerful instruments, they are also difficult to control with any degree of precision. As a consequence, incentives are likely to give rise to unplanned and unwanted side effects. The trick that has yet to be discovered is how to use incentives in a way that promotes desired policy objectives without creating distortions elsewhere in the system. It is in this area, more than any other, that further work is needed to find the most effective way of reconciling cash-limited budgets with incentives that reward achievements. In this respect, the German system of paying doctors' fees, in which an overall cap on fees is combined with sliding scale payment systems, may warrant more study.

The Purchaser Role

It can be argued that one of the reasons the NHS reforms have not demonstrated greater benefits for patients so far is that the key role of health authorities as purchasers was given insufficient attention in the early stages of implementation. While steps have since been taken to strengthen the role of health authorities, a huge amount remains to be done to transform district health authorities from provider-oriented organisations to agencies which can become champions of the people. This is important because the raison d'être of the reforms is to move the NHS away from a history of provider dominance. The dominance of provider will only change if there is an effective countervailing force in a position to make an independent assessment of health needs, and allocate resources in response to those needs.

Early experience of the reforms showed that the purchaser role is only likely to develop effectively if there is a clear separation of purchaser and provider roles. In a situation in which district health authorities continue to carry ultimate responsibility for the performance of providers, it is difficult for purchasers to focus on the needs of the population rather than the demands of providers. This applies particularly to the ability of purchasers to improve health as well as health services. The agenda set out in *The Health of the Nation* will only be delivered if district health authorities are in a position to work with a range of agencies to tackle the conditions which give rise to avoidable mortality and morbidity. The attempt to refocus the attention of district health authorities on health rather than sickness will be hindered if providers are brought back under the control of district health authorities.

The best district health authorities are already demonstrating what it is possible to achieve using their new powers. This is illustrated in Box 10, which draws examples from a report published by the National Association of Health Authorities and Trusts. Of particular importance in this context is collaboration between district health authorities and family health services authorities. A study of collaboration published in 1993 (Ham, Schofield and Williams, 1993) illustrated the benefits resulting from joint commissioning in a number of leading-edge districts. This included the preparation of comprehensive health strategies and the higher priority given to primary care. One of the most significant conclusions of the study was that collaboration between district health authorities and family health services authorities had helped in the development of shared purchasing with GP fundholders. This was because district health authorities were able to benefit from the close relationships that family health services authorities had often established with GPs.

Box 10: The achievements of health authority purchasers.

In Dorset no one waits for over 6 months for elective in-patient surgery except in orthopaedics.

In Lewisham the out-patient waiting time for orthopaedics fell from 52 weeks to 6 weeks as a result of contracts being moved between providers.

In Scarborough physiotherapy waiting times were reduced from 20 weeks to 3 weeks as a result of evening clinics in hospitals and GP surgeries.

In Leicestershire a major investment was made to increase open access services for GPs, including an extension of radiology, ultrasound and physiotherapy.

In the Wirral, termination of pregnancy services contracts were renegotiated to enable these services to be provided in the district rather than outside.

Source: NAHAT (1993)

The challenge is to build on this experience and to coordinate effectively the decisions of fundholders. This will help to avoid the instability which will occur if fundholders and district health authorities operate independently. One way of achieving this would be to channel the budgets of fundholders through health authorities and make them conditional on GPs signing up to local health strategies developed by health authorities. In this way, it is possible to see how a coherent purchasing function could develop enabling national policies, like *The Health of the Nation*, to be taken forward on a consistent basis and ensuring proper accountability of fundholders.

Management

In emphasising the role of contestability, incentives and purchasers, it is important not to neglect the contribution of effective management to the delivery of health services. As we have noted, this is fundamental to health care reform in a number of countries and it continues to be a significant factor within the NHS. The *Griffiths Report* of 1983 was a watershed in the management of the NHS and in many ways it laid the foundations for the reforms contained in *Working for Patients*. As a result of these publications there was a significant increase in the number of managers working in the NHS and a profound change in working style. General managers have played a major part in delivering the government's policies in the last decade and it was therefore all the more ironic that the increase in management costs should be attacked from within the government.

The plans announced by Ministers during 1993 to reorganize the structure of the NHS and streamline management arrangements were motivated largely by concern that as much of the NHS budget as possible is spent on direct patient care (Department of Health, 1993c). While this is a laudable objective, it has to be recognized that the NHS is a vast organization demanding effective management. It is essential therefore to distinguish those areas where savings can be made without affecting patient care and those areas where a crude attack on management costs is likely to be counterproductive.

During 1993 it was estimated that around 12,000 staff were employed above the level of local management in regional health authorities, the NHS management executive and the Department of Health (Ham, 1993b). This figure is likely to fall significantly as a result of the proposals contained in *Managing the New NHS*. Although detailed plans have yet to be published, it is widely accepted that the central management of the NHS needs to adapt its role in line with the changes that have taken place among purchasers and providers. The result will be a small, head office function in the NHS executive supported by slimline regional offices and a Department of Health whose functions and responsibilities are commensurate with these changes. There is little doubt that these reforms are much needed and represent a belated attempt by those at the centre to catch up with developments within the NHS.

At the local level of management, the proposed merger of district health authorities and family health services authorities, together with a continuing reduction in the number of district health authorities, will also help to cut down duplication and free up resources for patient services. Beyond this it is difficult to identify areas in which savings can be made when it remains government policy to expand the GP fund-holding scheme (with its associated management costs) and to strengthen the role of purchasers. If the policy pursued in Wales of setting an arbitrary limit on management costs is followed in England, there is a risk that purchasers will be hamstrung in their efforts to bring about improvements in health and health services. It is particularly at this point in the NHS that good management is most needed and where too stringent controls may prevent managers from carrying out their responsibilities effectively.

One way of squaring the circle would be to pursue a policy of contestability rather than competitive tendering. Part of the increase in management costs is a consequence of the transaction costs involved in a contract system. Some of these costs could be avoided if purchasers and providers worked together in long term, collaborative relationships, resorting to tendering for contracts only when other approaches fail to improve performance. To this extent, Ministers may have to choose between a more competitive approach with higher transaction costs and the philosophy of contestability, which is more efficient to administer but which may bring fewer benefits in the longer term.

However this argument is resolved, management arrangements among purchasers and providers will continue to change rapidly as the reforms are implemented. For providers, this will involve a further strengthening of clinical management. Clinical directorates (or their equivalents) will become the building blocks around which the organization is shaped and the level of management support within directorates will be enhanced. This will enable clinicians to play a more effective part in contract negotiations and it will help to establish a direct dialogue between directorates and the purchasers of their services. It follows that the top management team will have a key role in coordinating activities in different directorates as well as providing leadership for the organization as a whole. Reflecting trends in organizations across both the public and private sectors (Peters, 1992; Handy, 1989), middle managers will increasingly disappear as these arrangements are put in place and as the function of directorates is strengthened. One of the benefits of this approach will be to develop greater clinical ownership of contracts, thereby avoiding some of the difficulties that arise when providers have over performed.

As far as purchasers are concerned, the gradual transformation of district health authorities from provider dominated agencies to purchasers has already brought about a change of approach and attitudes. The organizations that have been created to support purchasing contain far fewer staff than the old style district health authorities and most of their staff hold senior positions in functions such as public health, finance, planning and contracting. Further changes can be anticipated as district health authorities engage in joint commissioning with family health services authorities, and as some of the functions involved in purchasing are bought in rather then being provided in-house.

One of the weaknesses of the district health authority model of purchasing is that citizens are not able to choose which authority purchases services on their behalf as this is determined by place of residence. To overcome this, and to introduce a degree of contestability into purchasing, it has been suggested that the management of purchasing organizations could be opened up to competitive forces (Ham, 1993e). If this were to happen, the job of the chairman and non-executive directors would be to determine who should take on this role for a given period of time. There are precedents of this kind in relation to public education services in the United States (Hodges, 1993) and proposals have recently been put forward to make public institutions contestable in the United Kingdom (Mulgan, 1993). If this were to happen, it would open up the possibility of competition for the management of purchasing organizations among agencies with a range of characteristics, some offering skills in contract management and negotiation, others bringing expertise in relation to needs' assessment and public participation.

70

Accountability

Working for Patients took the changes brought about by the 1983 *Griffiths Report* a stage further by introducing a unitary board for NHS authorities and trusts. This entails a small number of non-executive directors sitting alongside their executive colleagues (*see* Box 11). As part of this change, many of the chairmen and non-executive directors on the new boards were appointed from outside the NHS, often bringing with

Box 11: The composition of the new health authorities.

	Family Health Services Authority	Regional Health Authority	District Health Authority	NHS Trust
Chairman Appointed by	Secretary of State	Secretary of State	Secretary of State	Secretary of State
Non-executives on the authority	Five lay members appointed by Regional Health Authority, four professional members appointed by Regional Health Authority	Five appointed by Secretary of State including a Family Health Services Authority chairman and a member who holds a post in a university with a medical or dental school	Five appointed by Regional Health Authority – teaching districts to include a member who holds a post in a university with a medical or dental school	Up to five including at least two appointed from local community by Regional Health Authority – rest to be appointed by Secretary of State including a person from the relevant medical school where a trust has teaching responsibilities
Executives on the authority	Chief executive	Up to five including chief executive and finance director	Up to five including chief executive and finance director	Up to five including chief executive, finance director, medical director, senior nurse

them experience of business and commerce. This brought a number of benefits in terms of a more corporate way of working and a sharper approach to decision making. However, in a few cases NHS boards acted outside their powers and wasted significant sums of public money.

It was in response to these developments that the Secretary of State set up a task force on corporate governance in the NHS during 1993. The task force noted in particular the difficulties that had arisen in the Wessex and West Midlands Regional Health Authorities in formulating its proposals. These proposals emphasized the need for there to be accountability, probity and openness within the NHS. The task force set out a code of conduct and a code of accountability for the NHS and recommended that the boards of health authorities and trusts should establish audit and remuneration committees of their non-executive directors. The need for chairmen and non-executives to have training and support to enable them to carry out their responsibilities was also emphasized.

The report of the corporate governance task force served as an important reminder that the introduction of techniques drawn from the private sector had to be done in a way that was sensitive to the requirements of the public sector. It also raised questions about the composition of NHS boards and arrangements for ensuring accountability. The unitary boards introduced in 1990 may have been more businesslike than their predecessors but they involve fewer people drawn from local communities and, in the case of NHS trusts, were required to hold only one public meeting a year. Arguments that a new magistracy (Stewart, 1992) was emerging to run public services found plenty of supporting evidence within the NHS. These arguments also served to highlight the democratic deficit at a local level in the new NHS.

One response to this was to argue for greater democratic control over the running of the NHS. This cut little ice with the government. While recognizing the need for health authorities and trusts to be accountable to their communities, Ministers stopped short of suggesting that this should be achieved by elected health authorities or by giving local government a bigger say in the organization of health services. Rather, they underlined the role of community health councils in speaking on behalf of local people and enjoined health authorities and trusts to be open and accessible in the way they conducted their affairs.

These issues assumed greater significance as health authorities, in their new purchasing guise, responded to the challenge of setting priorities and rationing scare resources. A study of how district health authorities were approaching priority setting suggested that four sets of influences were particularly important (Ham, Honigsbaum and Thompson, 1994). On the vertical axis, national and regional 'givens' and the views of local professionals had been the key factors at work in the old NHS and continued to be important (see Figure 11). These influences were combined with the views of the public and evidence of cost and effectiveness, represented on the horizontal axis. It was argued that the public's views and evidence of cost and effectiveness might exert greater influence as district health authorities gained confidence in their purchasing role and took a more critical view of the claims emanating from providers.

The study also found that district health authorities were using a variety of methods to involve the public in decision making on priorities. These methods included undertaking questionnaire surveys, consulting with community groups and voluntary organisations, and working with community health councils. One of the reasons why district health authorities were seeking to involve the public was recognition that priority setting could not be reduced to a technical or scientific exercise. Given the need to make judgements about priorities, it was argued that these judgements were likely to be more soundly based and defensible if they had been exposed to public discussion. Put slightly differently, given that

Figure 11: Pressures on purchasing authorities.

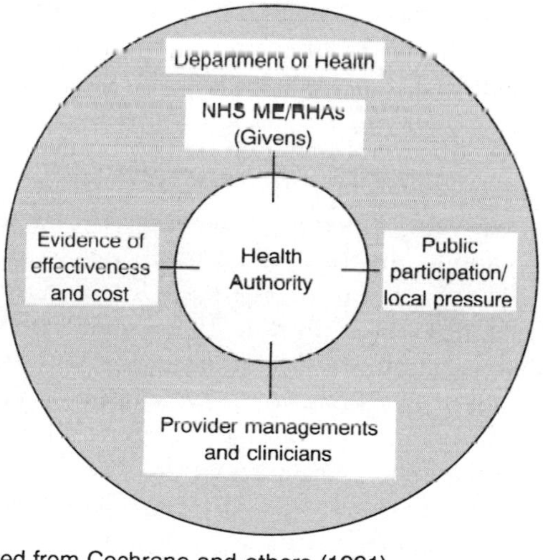

Source: Adapted from Cochrane and others (1991)

there was no right answer in the priority setting debate, an important justification for the decisions made was that they had been arrived as a result of due process.

This was easier said than done. Research into public participation in decision making on priorities indicated that it was often difficult to generate interest on the part of the public and the public's view were influenced critically by the methods used (Bowling and others, 1993). These findings reinforced the notion put forward by the Secretary of State for Health that there needed to be greater 'health literacy' if the population was to participate fully in decisions on resource allocation (Department of Health, 1993b).

Primary Care

One of the most significant benefits of the NHS reforms is the renewed emphasis on primary care. In view of the origins of the reforms in a crisis in the acute hospital services, this requires some explanation. In part, it has resulted from the priority given to the reform of primary care by Kenneth Clarke, and in part is stemmed from the shift in the balance of power brought about by *Working for Patients*. The effect has been to consolidate the already pivotal position of GPs and primary care teams within the NHS and to move resources and services in the direction of primary care. GP fundholders have been in the vanguard of these developments and their interest has been matched by many district health authorities and family health services authorities, who have pursued a policy in which priority has been given to primary care-led purchasing of secondary care.

As the reforms go forward, it will be important to maintain the momentum generated in this area. On this point, the signals from within the NHS are contradictory. On the one hand, there is a great deal of energy and enthusiasm in many places as primary care climbs higher up the policy agenda. On the other hand, there are indications that morale in some parts of general practice is low and that a significant number of GPs resent the administrative burden imposed by the 1990 contract. Fundholding has acted as a divisive influence in this context, polarising opinion among GPs and creating strong feelings on all sides.

Against this background, it is essential that the strengths of primary care within the NHS are not dissipated. At one level, this involves continuing to take action to improve the poorest standards of primary care, whether these are found in inner cities or elsewhere. At another level, it entails responding to the legitimate concern of GPs about unnecessary paperwork and excessive workload. Plans already under discussion to end GPs' round-the-clock commitment will provide some assistance in this respect but a broader programme is needed encompassing the terms under which GPs work within the NHS.

The outcome may well be a greater variety of contractual arrangements for GPs. This could include the option of salaried employment as well as independent contractor status, a development already happening in some parts of the NHS. It may also mean moving away from a national contract to an arrangement in which health authorities have discretion at a local level to negotiate with GPs for the provision of certain services. These services will include not only general medical services as traditionally understood but a wider range of primary and social care. As this happens, the role of nurses and paramedical staff in primary care will be further enhanced.

The scope of things to come is illustrated by development in Dorset where the Health Commission (an agency which brings together the district health authority and family health services authority) has been working hand in hand with primary care teams to explore new ways of delivering services. In one initiative, two GP practices in Lyme Regis are collaborating in the provision of a range of community health services from a primary care base. In another initiative, a large fundholding practice in Swanage offers an extended range of services in association with an NHS trust and under contract to the Health Commission (Ham, Schofield and Williams, 1993). The point about both initiatives is that they involve collaboration between primary care teams and health authorities and a switch of resources towards primary care to enable services to be delivered in this way. It is this emphasis on the provision of services in primary care that is at least as important as the debate about GPs as purchasers.

In the broader context, the devolution of services and resources to primary care must be matched by accountability for the use of those resources. Family health services authorities in some parts of the NHS have made a start in this area by undertaking annual reviews of primary care teams and setting standards for the improvement of services. Publication of a *Patient's Charter* for primary care is a move in the same direction. With reaccreditation of GPs under active discussion, there is a real opportunity to bring general practice into the mainstream of the

NHS – provided that this is done sensitively and respects a proper degree of autonomy for GPs.

There is much greater uncertainty over the future of dental and pharmaceutical services administered by family health services authorities. General dental practitioners in many parts of the country declined to provide a service to adult patients within the NHS because of dissatisfaction with the contract introduced in 1990. In response, the government set up an independent review under Sir Kenneth Bloomfield and this identified a number of options for the future. At the time of writing, the government's reaction to the Bloomfield report is awaited. Meanwhile patients who are unable to obtain NHS dental care are required to pay for private treatment. Family health services authorities have been given greater responsibility for the payment of pharmacists, particularly where they provide additional professional services. This means a move away from a fee structure based mainly on the number of prescriptions dispensed by pharmacists, towards renumeration based in part on their professional skills. In the case of both pharmacists and dentists, there is therefore likely to be greater local discretion over contracts and payments in the future, and the same principles may well be extended to GPs.

Strategy

More important than any of the issues discussed so far is the direction in which the reforms are taking the NHS. The changes contained in *Working for Patients* were primarily about means rather than ends. In a manner that has become familiar within British politics, having decided on the means the government then turned its attention to the ends it wished to pursue. The outcome was the publication of the *Patient's Charter* and the national health strategy, *The Health of the Nation*. In addition, Ministers have pursued a large number of other policy initiatives. The result has been to overload the health policy agenda and to create the impression of a lack of vision at the highest level. As we noted earlier, the reason behind this is the rapidly changing stewardship of the NHS among Secretaries of State and Prime Ministers and the tendency to pile one policy initiative on top of others.

In relation to the NHS reforms, tactics have come to dominate strategy. This has served the interests of Ministers in the short term by keeping the NHS out of the headlines and reducing the level of critical comment directed at government policy but it has created a vacuum for the NHS as a whole. While it would be naive to believe that the NHS will ever operate within a clearly defined framework involving a limited number of neatly ordered priorities, it is incumbent on Ministers (of whatever party) to provide a sense of direction to those purchasing and providing services on their behalf. Put simply, where are the reforms taking the NHS and what is the purpose of the NHS now and in the future?

In developing a strategy for the NHS, Ministers should begin by reviewing the founding principles of 1948 and assess whether they remain relevant. As we have noted on several occasions, equity and access, two of the key founding principles, have come under pressure as the NHS market has placed greater emphasis on efficiency and responsiveness. Despite this, Ministers continue to reassert their commitment to the basis on which the NHS was established and argue that their support for the NHS is unwavering.

The reality is that so much has changed since 1948 that the assumptions on which the NHS was based do need to be reexamined. The result may well be acceptance that it is worth sacrificing a degree of equity (for example, by allowing fundholders to negotiate quicker access to hospitals for their patients) in the pursuit of other values. This can only be determined by an honest reappraisal of the purpose of the NHS as we approach the end of the century and its role alongside other forms of provision. Such a reappraisal should not be confined to health services but must assess the wider influences on health, for example poverty, housing and employment opportunities.

Nowhere does this apply with greater force than in relation to the founding principle of comprehensiveness. In theory, the NHS is supposed to provide comprehensive services to all citizens, although when individuals have taken legal action to enforce this right it has emerged that the Secretary of State has a large measure of discretion in deciding which service can be provided within the available resources. And in practice, the scope of the NHS has been narrowed by a series of incremental decisions affecting optical services, adult dentistry and long-term nursing care. While this has succeeded in minimising political turbulence (tactics dominating strategy again), it hardly represents an approach that can be sustained in the long term. Furthermore, the decision by the Ombudsman that the NHS has an obligation to provide nursing care to patients who are seriously ill seems certain to intensify the debate about explicit rationing.

A more defensible policy would be to acknowledge that the NHS cannot do everything and to initiate an open discussion about future priorities. To pass this responsibility entirely to district health authorities runs the risk of further undermining equity, as different authorities come up with different lists of priorities. In a situation in which resources will always be limited, political honesty needs to go hand in hand with health literacy in a public debate about the principles of rationing and priority setting.

Given the work going into the government's fundamental review of public expenditure, it can only be a matter of time before these issues receive the prominence they deserve. The language of strategy, principles, and priorities is (or ought to be) the language of politics. The fact that they have been neglected in recent times does not make them any less important. While there are those who will no doubt argue that government policy has been driven by an implicit strategy since 1989 (our old friend the hidden agenda of privatization), this is taking conspiracy theories beyond the bounds of credibility. Not only are governments not that clever, but also it would be electoral suicide for any government to undermine the NHS, however surreptitiously. The absence of a coherent strategy reflects a deeper malaise in British politics and one which encompasses opposition parties as well as those in government. In these circumstances, the party or politicians that can articulate a credible vision can lay claim to the most valued prize of all.

Conclusion

The future of the NHS remains uncertain. In the light of experience gained since 1991, it is possible to see how the NHS reforms might be taken forward to the benefit of patients and the public. This requires a more explicit policy of market management, an emphasis on contestability rather than competition, the more imaginative use of budgetary incentives, greater support for the role of purchasers, recognition of the need for effective management at a local level, a stronger emphasis on accountability, and support for the development of primary care. Above all, politicians must grasp the nettle of strategy and determine how the various means contained within the reforms can be used to create a new NHS fit to enter the 21st century.

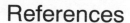

References

Bowling, A. and others (1993) Health services priorities: explorations in consultation of the public and health professionals on priority setting in an inner London health district, *Social Science and Medicine*, 37, 7, 851–7.

Bloor, K. and Maynard, A. (1993) *Expenditure on the NHS during and after the Thatcher years*. Centre for Health Economics, University of York.

Bradlow, J. and Coulter, A. (1993) Effect of fundholding and indicative prescribing scheme on general practitioners' prescribing costs, *British Medical Journal*, 307, 1186–9.

Brindle, D. (1993a) Dangerous time for a famous name, *The Guardian*, 28 July.

Brindle, D. (1993b) Casualties in a war of words, *The Guardian*, 20 October.

Clinical Standards Advisory Group (1993) *Access to and availability of specialist services*. HMSO, London.

Cochrane, M. and others (1991) Rationing: at the cutting edge, *British Medical Journal*, 303, 1039–42.

Coulter, A. (1992) Fundholding general practices, *British Medical Journal*, 304, 397–8.

Department of Health (1993a) *Virginia Bottomley reaffirms commitment to the underlying principles of the NHS*. DoH, London (press release).

Department of Health (1993b) *Virginia Bottomley calls for greater openness in NHS decision making*. DoH, London (press release).

Department of Health (1993c) *Managing the new NHS*. DoH, London.

Department of Health (1993d) *Making London better*. Health Publications Unit, Lancashire.

Eisenberg, J. (1986) *Doctors' decisions and the cost of medical care*. Health Administration Press, Ann Arbor.

Enthoven, A.C. (1985) *Reflections on the management of the NHS*. Nuffield Provincial Hospitals Trust, London.

Fowler, N. (1991) *Ministers decide* Chapman, London.

Glennerster, H. and others (1992) *A foothold for fundholding*. King's Fund Institute, London.

Ham, C. (1989) Clarke's strong medicine, *Marxism Today*, March, 38–41.

Ham, C. (1990a) *The new NHS*. Radcliffe Medical Press, Oxford.

Ham, C. (1990b) *Holding on while letting go*. King's Fund College, London.

Ham, C. (1990c) A picture of health, *Marxism Today*, July, 18–21.

Ham, C. (1991) Revisiting the internal market, *British Medical Journal*, 302, 250–1.

Ham, C. (1992a) *Health policy in Britain*. Macmillan, Basingstoke, 3rd edition.

Ham, C. (1992b) *Locality purchasing*. Health Services Management Centre, University of Birmingham.

Ham, C. (1992c) *Managed competition in the NHS: progress and prospects*. Manchester Statistical Society, Manchester.

Ham, C. (1992d) Growing pains of a difficult child, *The Guardian*, 5 September.

Ham, C. (1992e) Doctors' power, patients' risk, *The Guardian*, 25 March.

Ham, C. (1993a) How go the NHS reforms?, *British Medical Journal*, 306, 77–8.

Ham, C. (1993b) Reviewing the NHS review, *British Medical Journal*, 307, 5–6.

Ham, C. (1993c) The latest reorganisation of the NHS, *British Medical Journal*, 307, 1089–90.

Ham, C. (1993d) Health care reform, *British Medical Journal*, 306, 1223–4.

Ham, C. (1993e) Dial M for Management, *Health Service Journal*, April 1993.

Ham, C. and others (1989) *Managed competition*. King's Fund Institute, London.

Ham, C., Robinson, R. and Benzeval, M (1990) *Health check*. King's Fund Institute, London.

Ham, C. and Heginbotham, C. (1991) *Purchasing together*. King's Fund College, London.

Ham, C. and Haywood, S. (1992) *The NHS guide*. National Association of Health Authorities and Trusts, Birmingham.

Ham, C. Schofield, D. and Williams, J. (1993) *Partners in purchasing*. National Association of Health Authorities and Trusts, Birmingham.

Ham, C. Honigsbaum, F. and Thompson, D. (1994) *Priority setting for health gain*, Department of Health, London.

Ham, C. and Maynard, A. (1994) Managing the NHS Market, *British Medical Journal*, 308, 845–7.

Handy, C. (1989) *The age of unreason*. Business Books, London.

Hodges, L. (1993) Schools Inc takes charge, *The Independent*, 16 December.

IRS Employment Trends (1993) Local bargaining in the NHS: A survey of first and second wave trusts.

Laing, W. (1990) *Laing's review of private health care 1990/91*. Laing-Buisson Publications, London.

Lawson, N. (1992) *The view from No.11*. Bantam Press, London.

Ministry of Welfare, Health and Cultural Affairs (1992) *Choices in health care*. Rijswijk, The Ministry.

Mulgan, G. (1993) *The power of the boot: the case for contestable public institutions*. DEMOS, London.

NAHAT (1993) *NHS purchasing for a healthy population*. Birmingham.

National Advisory Committee (1992) *Core services 1993/4*. National Advisory Committee, Wellington.

NHSME (1989) *Role of district health authorities – analysis of issues*. London.

NHSME (1990) *Developing districts*. London.

NHSME (1991) *Assessing health care needs*. London.

NHSME (1992) *Local voices*. London.

OECD (1992) *The reform of health care: a comparative analysis of seven OECD countries*. OECD, Paris.

Peters, T. (1992) *Liberation management*. Macmillan, London.

Roberts, J. (1990) Kenneth Clarke: hatchet man or remoulder? *British Medical Journal*, 301, 1383–6.

Smith, R. (1991) William Waldegrave: thinking beyond the new NHS, *British Medical Journal*, 302, 711–4.

Stewart, J. (1992) *The rebuilding of public accountability*. Paper presented to the European Policy Forum.

Timmins, N. (1993) GP to refuse 'costly' patients, *The Independent*, 9 October.

Tomlinson Report (1992) *Report of the inquiry into London's health service, medical education and research*. HMSO, London

Index